## Praise for *Embodied Resilie*

"A much-needed addition to any yoga book collection, providing an uninhibited voice to many powerful leaders who teach the reader important lessons about humanity, compassion, and how yoga helps us be and do better."

—Jules Mitchell, author *Yoga Biomechanics: Stretching Redefined*

"Through the medium of hard-earned stories, this diverse collection of essays invites the reader to ask foundational questions about embodied resilience: What do I carry? What can I let go of? What am I ready to heal? And finally, how can yoga help? These authentic writing voices also deftly explore the intersection between personal experiences and transformative action. They offer a roadmap for facilitating social change from inside-to-out."

—Matthew Sanford, author of *Waking: A Memoir of Trauma and Transcendence*, yoga teacher, and founder of the non-profit Mind Body Solutions

"When you've experienced trauma, the journey home to the body can be challenging at best. These incredible stories illustrate how yoga that's taught and practiced in a way that helps you gently tune your ear to your body and inner knowing can be a powerful companion on the way."

—Anna Guest-Jelley, founder of Curvy Yoga

"This book shares personal stories that demonstrate how yoga can be the missing link in healing from trauma and building resilience. It shares the experiences of what it means to be in the yoga space and be fat, transgender, or person of color. It also shows what it is like to come to yoga when working through an eating disorder, drug addiction, or grief. By reading this book, the reader becomes aware of and learns about perspectives that they might not otherwise know of due to privilege or having different life experiences. It acts as a powerful tool not just to foster awareness of larger social issues, but also to promote discussions."

—Trina Altman, NCPT, E-RYT 500, YACEP®

"The stunning beauty and power of the collected essays in *Embodied Resilience through Yoga* are found not only in the liberating diversity of voices, but in the ability of narrative to foster empathy and inclusion. They all highlight, in rich and varied ways, the value of yoga as a means to healing and empowerment—not in some obtuse, mystical way, but as a real and tangible tool for transformative change."

— Carrie Owerko, C-IAYT, Senior Intermediate Iyengar yoga teacher

"This book is embodiment itself: from beginning to end it honors the courage of vulnerability and deepens your relationship with yourself. Expect the shared humanity of pain, healing, and hope to resonate thoroughly in your body, and inspire the power within you."

—Dr. Jennifer Copeland, contemplative psychotherapist and yoga and meditation teacher

"Humanity has always used storytelling as the vehicle for teaching, and that's the beauty of this collection. We're offered essential teachings in the form of personal stories that get to the heart of the issues facing contemporary yoga practitioners. Read, reflect, repeat!"

—Jivana Heyman, author of *Accessible Yoga*

"Grateful, grateful, grateful. Thank you for this book; thank you for the truth it offers and the optimism it encourages."

—Jessamyn Stanley, author of *Every Body Yoga*

"Few things are more courageous than the re-imagining of our own narratives of resilience. As we move into post Covid-19, these intersectional stories of courage and hope are powerful mitigation during a time of collective trauma. With each story told and heard, maps are exchanged to help us all navigate our own hero's and heroine's journey into belonging and embodied resilience."

—Micheline Pierrette Berry, somatic artist and founder of Liquid Asana

"The inspirational stories of those who have used their traumatic experiences as sources of personal growth and community strength, along with the meditations and reflection questions that are included in *Embodied Resilience through Yoga*, serve as a much-needed healing balm."

—Gail Parker, PhD, CIAYT, author of *Restorative Yoga for Ethnic and Race-Based Stress and Trauma*

"*Embodied Resilience through Yoga* is exactly what we need to be reading right now to help us through these turbulent times and beyond."

—Anusha Wijeyakumar MA, RYT, CPC, founder of Shanti Within and wellness consultant at Hoag Hospital

"You will find yourself in these stories, and when you do, please take a breath, honor your own tender journey, and let the words on these pages remind you that although trauma runs deep, healing is possible and resiliency is a superpower that is found from within. The triumphs in these stories are not built on the wishes of magical thinking but earned from the hard work of turning inward for strength, compassion, and self-love. I highly recommend this beautiful book and am grateful to each author for sharing their truth so we can turn towards our own with more grace."

—Seane Corn, author of *Revolution of the Soul* and cofounder of Off the Mat, Into the World

"The editors and contributors of *Embodied Resilience through Yoga* prove that our personal stories can both inspire and educate. This vulnerable collection of essays offer insight into how yoga practice can be an avenue to healing and to living an embodied life. In moments when you need some motivation, amidst life's daily challenges, pick up and read or reread a bit of someone's truth to stay connected to your own."

—Felicia Tomasko, RN, editor-in-chief of *LA YOGA* magazine

"*Embodied Resilience through Yoga* is a well-written, must-read book for anyone who wants to discover the healing and transformational benefits of yoga."

—Donna Noble, MSc, yoga teacher and intuitive wellbeing coach *Yoga*

# EMBODIED RESILIENCE THROUGH YOGA

# About the Editors

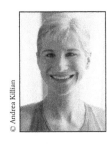

© Andrea Killian

**Kat Heagberg** is a writer, yoga teacher, and the editor in chief of Yoga International, an online platform dedicated to providing members with a diverse array of exclusive multimedia content for yoga, meditation, and mindful living. There, you can find her yoga classes, online courses, and articles. Kat's writing focuses on the power of language in yoga culture and creative ways to make yoga poses and practices more fun and accessible. She's the co-author of *Yoga Where You Are: Customize Your Practice for Your Body and Your Life* (Shambhala, 2020) with Dianne Bondy and the co-host of the *Yoga Talk* podcast with Kyle Rebar.

Visit her online at https://www.katdoeshandstands.com or on Instagram at @katheagberglar.

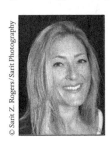

© Sarit Z. Rogers/Sarit Photography

**Melanie C. Klein, MA,** is an empowerment coach, thought leader, and influencer in the areas of body confidence, authentic empowerment, and visibility. She is also a successful writer, speaker, and professor of sociology and women's studies. Her areas of interest and specialty include media literacy education, body image, and the intersectional analysis of systems of power and privilege. She is the co-editor of *Yoga and Body Image: 25 Personal Stories About Beauty, Bravery & Loving Your Body* (Llewellyn, 2014) with Anna Guest-Jelley, a contributor in *21st Century Yoga: Culture, Politics, and Practice* (Kleio Books, 2012), is featured in *Conversations with Modern Yogis* (Confluence Pictures, 2014), a featured writer in *Llewellyn's Complete Book of Mindful Living* (Llewellyn, 2016), co-editor of *Yoga, the Body, and Embodied Social Change: An Intersectional Feminist Analysis* with Dr. Beth Berila and Dr. Chelsea Jackson Roberts (Rowman and Littlefield, 2016), and the editor of *Yoga Rising: 30 Empowering Stories from Yoga Renegades for Every Body* (Llewellyn, 2018). She co-founded the Yoga and Body Image Coalition in 2014 and lives in Santa Monica, CA.

Visit her online at melaniecklein.com or find her on Instagram at @melmelklein.

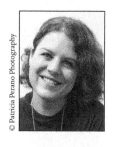

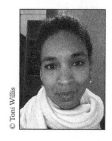

**Kathryn Ashworth** is a writer, editor, photographer, and yoga teacher with a background in anthropology. She views yoga as a healing resource that can awaken a sense of wonder and individual purpose, and her specific interests lie in simple and adaptable practices that anyone can benefit from. She currently works as an editor and yoga teacher at Yoga International.

**Toni Willis** lives in North Carolina where she writes fiction and edits books and web content, including articles for Yoga International. She enjoys yoga, vegan cooking, board games, and travel.

The practices and discussion questions included in this book were written by Michelle C. Johnson.

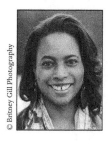

**Michelle C. Johnson** is a social justice warrior, author, dismantling racism trainer, empath, yoga teacher and practitioner, and an intuitive healer. Michelle has a bachelor of arts degree from the College of William and Mary and a master's degree in social work from the University of North Carolina at Chapel Hill. Michelle published *Skill in Action: Radicalizing Your Yoga Practice to Create a Just World* in 2017. She teaches workshops in yoga studios and community spaces nationwide. She is on the faculty of Off the Mat, Into the World, and she serves as the co-director of 18 Springs Healing Center in Winston-Salem, NC. Michelle was a TEDx speaker at Wake Forest University in 2019, and she has been interviewed on several podcasts in which she explores the premise and foundation of *Skill in Action*, creating ritual in justice spaces, our divine connection with nature and Spirit, and how we as a culture can heal. Visit her online at michellecjohnson.com.

KAT HEAGBERG, MELANIE C. KLEIN,
KATHRYN ASHWORTH & TONI WILLIS

# EMBODIED RESILIENCE THROUGH YOGA

30 Mindful Essays
About Finding Empowerment
After Addiction, Trauma,
Grief, and Loss

Llewellyn Publications
Woodbury, Minnesota

FIRST EDITION
First Printing, 2020

Cover design by Shira Atakpu
Cover photograph by Sarit Z Rogers

Llewellyn Publications is a registered trademark of Llewellyn Worldwide Ltd.

Library of Congress Cataloging-in-Publication Data
Names: Heagberg, Kat, author. | Klein, Melanie, author. | Ashworth, Kathryn
   R., author. | Willis, Toni, author.
Title: Embodied resilience through yoga : 30 mindful essays about finding
   empowerment after addiction, trauma, grief, and loss / Kat Heagberg,
   Melanie C. Klein, Kathryn Ashworth, Toni Willis.
Description: First edition. | Woodbury, Minnesota : Llewellyn Publications,
   2020. | Includes bibliographical references. | Summary: "This book
   features thirty personal essays of resilience found through yoga to
   support readers' healing journeys to find empowerment, connection, and
   growth following trauma. Authors tell stories of overcoming addiction,
   working through trauma, and learning how to heal from grief. This book
   presents essays that prove those experiences matter and that yoga can
   help people find the resilience to carry on. This book explores
   perspectives on trauma related to gender, identity, body image, and
   more"—Provided by publisher.
Identifiers: LCCN 2020016952 (print) | LCCN 2020016953 (ebook) | ISBN
   9780738762494 (paperback) | ISBN 9780738762869 (ebook)
Subjects: LCSH: Yoga—Therapeutic use. | Resilience (Psychology) | Psychic
   trauma—Alternative treatment. | Substance abuse—Alternative treatment.
Classification: LCC RM727.Y64 H43 2020 (print) | LCC RM727.Y64 (ebook) |
   DDC 613.7/046--dc23
LC record available at https://lccn.loc.gov/2020016952
LC ebook record available at https://lccn.loc.gov/2020016953

Llewellyn Publications
A Division of Llewellyn Worldwide Ltd.
2143 Wooddale Drive
Woodbury, MN 55125-2989
www.llewellyn.com

Printed in the United States of America

## Disclaimer

This book is not intended to provide medical advice or take the place of medical advice and treatment from your personal physician. Readers are advised to consult their doctors or other qualified health care professionals regarding the treatment of their medical problems. The publisher and the authors recommend common sense when contemplating the practices described in this work.

## Content Warning

Some of the essays in this book contain detailed descriptions of traumatic events including sexual assault, eating disorders, and domestic violence. Please use discretion and practice self-care when reading.

# Dedication

This book demanded a voice.

This book demanded the opportunity to serve as a platform for all the stories contained within.

This book is for everyone who's started the journey to healing.

This book is for everyone who's ready to begin the journey to healing.

This book is for everyone who doesn't (yet) know they're in need of healing.

Here's to those who've healed, those in the process of healing, those guiding and facilitating healing, and everyone and every body in need of healing.

May we support and uplift one another.

# Contents

# PART FOUR:
## EXPLORING THE INTERSECTION
## OF TRAUMA AND IDENTITY - 151

# PART FIVE:
## FAMILY AND BELONGING - 219

# Meditation List

# FOREWORD

## Hala Khouri

*Embodied Resilience through Yoga* is the third in a series of books born out of the Yoga and Body Image Coalition, whose mission is to change the face (and body) of yoga to promote a more inclusive image of what yoga is and who it is for. This book has a focus on healing from trauma. The writers all confront trauma in various forms and are able to use yoga as one tool to transform and heal. I don't know if we ever completely heal from trauma, but I do know that we can let ourselves be transformed by it for the better. This is what this book is about.

I read this whole book in one sitting—each story broke my heart open and wore away at the ball of cynicism that has formed over the past several years with the growing divide and trauma throughout our country. These are stories of resilience, perseverance, grit, and hope. The authors all worked really hard to heal, and, against many odds, succeeded. Their "success" did not come with a fairy tale ending—yoga did not save them; it was not the panacea that freed them from their pain forever. Yoga was a tool that helped them persevere and ride the ups and downs that are a normal part of healing. For some, yoga opened a door they never knew was there; for others, it offered a community of support, or it helped them find safety in their bodies for the first time ever.

For all of them, yoga facilitated a sense of acceptance that unlocked the door to their journey—acceptance of themselves, those who failed them, and the world, as well as acceptance of their own beauty, potential, and light.

I have dedicated much of my professional life to training yoga teachers to be trauma informed. I've been teaching yoga for twenty-five years, and I've been a trauma therapist and clinician in private practice for over a decade. I understand how vulnerable it can be for trauma survivors to walk into their first yoga class. Unresolved trauma can make the body feel like the enemy—sensations can be overwhelming or, the converse, dissociating from the body becomes the defense against feeling the intolerable. Healing from trauma is about reconnecting to the body so that it becomes a reliable ally rather than a burden to escape. It is also about normalizing our symptoms as an appropriate response to an overwhelming situation. Shame can often be our biggest barrier to healing.

The most cutting-edge trauma therapies have finally recognized that trauma lives in the body, not the mind. Until we can recalibrate the nervous system and move out of "fight-or-flight" or "shutdown" mode into a regulated state, talking about our trauma has limited effect. Yoga is one of the best tools for reconnecting to our sensations and releasing the energy associated with traumatic events and circumstances. For this reason, many of the folks in this book were able to be significantly helped by yoga even if it wasn't taught in a particularly trauma-informed way. It's a testament to our innate capacity to heal that so many of the writers could take the medicine that yoga can offer even if they were in spaces that weren't explicitly geared toward working with trauma.

Some of the writers share stories of dealing with systemic trauma like racism, transphobia, homophobia, and fatphobia. When the culture and systems at large harm us or don't see us, yoga can be a practice that helps us feel in control when there are larger things we can't control.

In essence, these are stories of post-traumatic growth. Stories of how the process of healing can be the catalyst to becoming our most authentic selves. Many of the authors share that the practice allowed them to feel worthy again and gave them the container to explore their body and psyche in a safe way. Others speak about community and compassionate teachers who gave them permission to rest and to be exactly who they are. Some speak of hating the practice at first but coming back to it because they knew it was helping them. All the stories are stories of re-membering—bringing back the lost parts of ourselves so we can be whole again.

My teacher, Peter Levine, says that although trauma is a fact of life, it doesn't have to be a life sentence. I always like to point out that trauma is not necessarily bad—it does not serve survivors to assume they are broken by the challenges they've had to endure. Rather, our traumas shape us. Just like a diamond is formed from a piece of coal that is bumped around, we are formed by the challenges that life puts in front of us. We are all diamonds of sorts—not perfect and shiny everywhere. Parts of us are broken, parts covered in coal, and parts as shiny as ever. This is wholeness: loving and including all the parts of ourselves and knowing that, in the end, we are all worthy, we all deserve to thrive, we all deserve love.

When we see ourselves in other people's stories, it can inspire us. I hope that as you read this anthology, you can let the stories that mirror your story give you hope and self-compassion and that the stories that aren't yours can help foster empathy and awareness. Empathy is a natural extension of self-compassion. The more we honor the broken and brilliant parts of ourselves, the more we can do that for others. This is the kind of world I want to live in. Stories like this can pave the way.

—Hala Khouri, MA, SEP, E-RYT
Cofounder, Off the Mat, Into the World

# INTRODUCTION

When *Yoga and Body Image: 25 Personal Stories About Beauty, Bravery & Loving Your Body* was released in 2014, it sparked necessary conversations about the ways that yoga practice and yoga culture can both help and harm our body image. It encouraged a critical examination of the ways we treat and talk about our bodies within the context of yoga. And for many of us, it led to a change in the way we teach or participate in yoga classes. It encouraged us to acknowledge the ways in which diet culture had seeped into yoga spaces and to reframe the ways that we promote yoga—not as a means for "fixing" our bodies, but rather as a tool for self-love, self-inquiry, and self-acceptance.

What we find particularly noteworthy is that what inspired these discussions and the changes they helped set in motion were *stories*. People sharing their lived experiences.

The follow-up, *Yoga Rising: 30 Empowering Stories from Yoga Renegades for Every Body*, furthered the conversation and kept the energy in motion, focusing even more on the intersection of body image, identity, and social justice.

As we saw the collective momentum that these first two anthologies generated continue to inspire discussion, we noticed some common themes arising—themes that we wanted to explore more fully on their own. And we heard stories from fellow yoga teachers and practitioners that we knew the yoga world needed to hear. We knew we needed to curate a third book of essays and that this book would focus specifically on the intersection of yoga, trauma, and resilience: embodied resilience through yoga.

## Acknowledging and Working with Trauma Within the Context of Yoga

Just as discussions about body image and social justice have become more prevalent in yoga spaces in recent years, so too have the topics of trauma and resilience. More and more organizations are offering trauma-informed teacher trainings, many yoga teachers and studios are adopting trauma-informed policies and practices (such as requiring consent for hands-on adjustments and using teaching language that is more invitational than authoritative), and yoga magazines and websites are highlighting the work of nonprofits focused on addressing trauma.

In addition to recognizing that, as human beings, *many* of us who show up to yoga class likely have some experience with trauma, there's a growing conversation, both in and outside of the yoga world, about the role embodiment and mindfulness practices have to play in working with and healing from trauma, addiction, grief, and loss. In other words, about how these tools can help us move from trauma to *resilience*: our innate ability to heal and grow and thrive in the midst of adversity.

Though the intersection of yoga, trauma, and resilience isn't about a quick fix, and yoga is not a substitute for professional medical care, for many, its practices have served as tools for self-reflection, self-connection, and healing. This book is about sharing those experiences.

## At the Heart of This Conversation Reside Our Individual Stories

Though resilience has become a hot topic in yoga and mindfulness circles, trauma is still often discussed as though it is something that affects "other people," despite it being a common human experience. As a result, those who have experienced trauma and who live with its effects often feel othered in yoga, meditation, and movement spaces. That's why we think a book like this is so needed: representation.

Perhaps within these pages you might recognize yourself, your loved ones, your yoga students. Perhaps you might also realize that the experiences of others are very different from your own—and that's one reason why sharing our stories is so powerful: They give us a glimpse into the lives of others. They allow us access to experiences that are unlike our own—experiences that we ourselves may never have been aware of, but experiences that we *must* pay attention to if we are to cultivate positive, lasting change.

It is our hope that the essays in this book spark not only discussion but *action*. That the shared experiences of the authors—who include yoga practitioners, yoga teachers, mental health professionals, and activists—will pave the way for yoga spaces that are more trauma informed, inclusive, welcoming, and kind. And that they will remind us that the gift of embodiment is coupled with the gift of resilience—that within us *all* lies the capacity to learn and to grow. While our experiences are different, our humanity is shared.

Kat, Melanie, Kathryn, and Toni

# PART ONE

## *Trauma, Addiction, and Recovery*

Anyone who has been either directly or indirectly affected by addiction knows it can come in many forms, including addictions to substances such as alcohol or drugs and addictions to specific activities or behaviors. Addiction can even take the form of a compulsive relationship to yoga. However painful this coping mechanism may be, and harmful in the long term, addiction often gives us a sense of control during times in our lives that feel unmanageable. It is often the tool we have when there is no other. In this section, we witness a raw and humanistic exploration of these coping mechanisms and the journey we take as individuals toward finding other, more life-affirming resources.

Jan Adams struggled to feel a sense of belonging from an early age, and when her mother died from suicide, it only exacerbated that problem. In the years that followed, she found various means for numbing out and forgetting—from alcohol to drugs, to disordered eating and exercise addiction. But after finding the 12-step program, her relationship to a higher power, and yoga, she learned to make unconscious memories conscious and enter a loving relationship with her mind and her body.

Nicole Lang knew she was an alcoholic from the first sip of alcohol she took. She was twelve, and it was how she coped with the divorce of her parents and the depression she felt. In later years, after more trauma, including sexual assault, she started doing drugs and began engaging in acts of self-harm. But through a mix of academia and yoga she found sobriety, establishing a positive connection to her body by facing her traumas and releasing stored emotions.

In his essay, Colin Hall takes a deep dive into asana addiction, exploring how the cultural notion that being a good person means being a hardworking person often affects how we approach the practice of yoga. He explores this topic through the lens of social theory, history, and his own personal history as the "hardworking yogi." He also offers suggestions for practitioners who feel a desire to reevaluate the role this practice plays in their life.

Finding yoga helped Jill Weiss Ippolito recover her life after heroin addiction, and it also introduced her to a newfound purpose: what would become UpRising yoga (of which she is the founder). Knowing that yoga saved her life, she now offers the gifts of this practice by making it both affordable and accessible to incarcerated youth and underserved communities. In her own words, "We all can reach out and offer whatever we can in order to help ease the suffering of another. I'm grateful to pass this message along and to inspire others to do the same."

When David Holzer found yoga, he found community and a safe haven that would help him transition into a sober lifestyle. He became more awake to the feelings he had, including the grief he felt over the loss of his longtime partner. Though originally he felt like a "wolf among swans" in studio spaces, he eventually realized that he was not alone in his trauma, that those he practiced alongside also had their stories to tell. His story is a powerful reminder that we are always stronger when we acknowledge our togetherness.

*Each of the five parts of this book begins with a meditation and journaling practice from Michelle C. Johnson intended to help you prepare for and integrate the essays that follow. Explore the practices before or after reading each section and anytime in your life that they feel useful.*

# MEDITATION

---

## *Still and Quiet Enough to Listen*

We will start with a breathing practice to quiet your mind.

Find a comfortable seat or, if you prefer, you can stand or lie down.

To find a comfortable seat, you might want to elevate your hips by sitting on a cushion, pillow, or blanket.

Close your eyes or look at the ground in front of you and begin to breathe into your body. Start by taking deep breaths in and out. Begin to notice what moves in your body as you breathe. Notice all the parts of your body that move as you breathe.

Begin to notice the waves of breath as they begin and end.

Now, continue to breathe and begin to match the length of your inhale and exhale. This is equal-part breathing and can help with clarity and quieting the mind.

Sit for at least three minutes practicing equal-part breathing.

Notice the physical sensations and the emotions.

Embrace what you notice.

Now bring your awareness back to the breath and be still and quiet and listen. Listen as you sit quietly to what is beyond your mind and thoughts. Listen to what is at the core of who you are and embrace what you hear.

Embrace what you notice.

Emotions may arise; allow them to be present as you sit quietly and listen. See what you hear.

Once you feel ready to move out of meditation, with each breath cycle bring your awareness back to your body and the physical sensations that are present. Return to the space by opening your eyes.

—Michelle C. Johnson

# I AM A SURVIVOR

## *Jan Adams*

My gran Freda used to say that what doesn't kill you makes you stronger. I thought she was full of crap but today, I know she was right. I am who I am because of what I have survived. I am a fierce, loving, joyful, kind, and compassionate woman. I am a survivor.

I was born and raised in a small Canadian town. My family looked like any other nuclear family in the 1960s. My mum was an activist, and she instilled in me a social conscience, enlisting my help in her many social justice efforts, demanding that I see the world beyond my idyllic little Canadian town. My parents believed in science, that religion and God were for fools. I was taught that humans, the pinnacle of evolution, were the masters of the universe. If I were to succeed, I had to depend on myself.

I can't explain why but I always felt like an outsider, especially within my family. I believed that inside me lived an awful monster, terrified that if anyone glimpsed the real me, they would be horrified. I was lonely and sad but learned very early on how to pretend I was like other kids. I lived with a knot in my gut, on guard not to let my mask slip. At home I protected myself with my best friend, my blanket Quigley. At night I would suck my thumb and hum myself to sleep. My mum tried to stop me by painting an awful-tasting liquid on my thumb. I quickly learned that if I could endure the nasty taste for a few minutes I could happily suck my thumb all night.

## Implosion

My family imploded when I was twelve. On a sunny day in October 1975, my mum killed herself. I remember that day like it was yesterday; the clear blue sky, the people crowded into our house, the sad looks in their eyes. I never felt worthy of her love, and perhaps because I was old enough to understand what had happened, but not wise enough to know I couldn't have changed things, I believed I was the reason she took her life. The day before she died, I walked in on my mum as she was writing the letters she left us and for many years believed I could have saved her if I'd only paid more attention. I still have her letter, safe behind my favorite photo of us. Each time I read her words, different parts stand out to me. Today, I know she loved me very much and took her life in an attempt to give me a better one. I have been in the same dark place in my life many times, and each time I wanted to die I'd have a sense of her telling me not to do it. I'd feel her telling me that somewhere in my life was a moment of joy, and that if I killed myself, I'd miss it.

I was told to pretend Mum had gone away on a trip and was never coming back. That lie instilled in me the power of denial. For the next fifteen years nobody ever spoke about my mum or her suicide. It was as if she'd never existed. I felt I had to carry this shameful secret and would betray my family if I ever spoke about it.

The night my mum died, to help me sleep, my gran gave me a cup of hot milk laced with brandy. It smelled bad, and I didn't want to drink it, but she assured me it would make me feel better. I plugged my nose and chugged it back. I can still feel the heat of that drink spreading through my chest. I no longer felt like the horrible monster child who'd driven her mum to suicide. I had three cups of hot milk that night! Alcohol was a magic elixir that took away my worries and fears. I was instantly hooked. Just like the nasty paint on my thumb, I realized that if I could ignore the horrible taste, I would be rewarded.

I believe I was born an addict. It began with alcohol, but if I could use anything to alter my mood, I would. I had been trying to change my feelings and thoughts my entire life, and in alcohol, and later drugs, I found what I thought was freedom from the bondage of myself.

Alcohol and drugs gave me the courage to be someone else, the power to forget. I used as often as I could, and within a very short time, I knew I had lost control, doing things I was ashamed of. But I couldn't live without using because if I was not getting high, I was thinking about killing myself. I felt trapped in a vicious cycle, sure I would end up like my mum. Often that thought was comforting because suicide would be a final solution to my pain.

I was a strong, coordinated girl, successful in many sports. I also secretly felt that my body was the enemy. I felt ashamed of my body and was disgusted by any feelings I experienced. I desperately wanted someone, anyone, to love me but felt dirty and ashamed when anyone gave me a compliment or showed interest in me.

## Switching Addictions

At sixteen I joined the swim team and decided to quit using. Being a star athlete was more acceptable than being a drunk, and swimming gave me a new way to numb out. I'd dive into the pool and drown my feelings by pushing myself to exhaustion. I loved the feeling of controlling my body with exercise. Within months I developed an eating disorder. I had two dominating thoughts: when I felt I was bad or not good enough, I would binge and throw up, and when I felt someone hurt me, I would starve myself.

I swam throughout university and was prescribed sleeping pills because I was so undernourished and sick that my muscles were constantly twitching, but when I looked in the mirror, I saw a fat girl. When people expressed concern about my weight, my mind twisted their words, convincing me skinny meant lovable.

My life was controlled by my need to numb out, and I utilized a variety of compulsive behaviors to control all aspects of my life. I knew that when I drank I had no control and would do things I'd regret. I also knew that when all my other addictions failed, I could rely on alcohol.

I could manage for a while, but I'd eventually feel my only options were drinking or suicide. Thankfully, I always chose drinking. On the outside I appeared successful, but inside I still felt like the horrible monster child who drove her mum to suicide.

## Speaking My Truth

My life changed again on Christmas Day 1989. Stumbling drunk past my childhood home, I knew I was in trouble, still that lost little girl who believed she was unlovable. For the first time, I told my best friend about my mum's death, about how I really felt. I don't know why I chose that time and place to speak my truth, but I do know it was the beginning of my transformation from victim to survivor. I had no idea what to do, but I knew something had to change or I would die.

When I hit bottom, the hand of recovery was waiting for me. Two good friends attended 12-step programs, and through them I was introduced to a new way of living. I had used many addictions to manage my life and had to learn new skills if I was going to live joyfully.

One blessing of recovery is that I found a Higher Power and a sense of hope. I had long believed my mum's suicide was proof that God did not exist, that I was alone on this journey. I believed I couldn't trust people because they'd ultimately hurt me. In recovery I learned to take risks and trust others, to face life on life's terms. I began to talk about my feelings and thoughts and to let go of some of the pain I carried inside. The knot in my stomach started to dissolve, and I began to feel safe letting down my mask. I came to believe that I am a beautiful child of the universe.

I was sober but continued to use food and exercise to manage my feelings and thoughts. I looked good on the outside but was still struggling. It was easy to be abstinent from alcohol and drugs, but I had to eat to survive. Recovery from food and exercise addiction was harder because I continually had to monitor my relationships with these addictions. Was I eating to stuff my feelings or starving to kill them? Was I exercising to stay fit or to avoid my feelings? I still clung to the belief that I could look good on the outside without letting go of all my addictions.

## Memories Crash In

Early in sobriety, my life fell apart when vivid memories of being sexually abused throughout my childhood smashed through the thick walls of denial I had built around these events. I trusted my Higher Power would only give me what I could handle and believed that no matter how bad these memories were I would survive. Though the memories brought tremendous pain, they were the catalyst that helped me begin to heal the twisted relationship I had with my body.

In early recovery, I was afraid to have sex, fearing I'd relapse. When I finally did have sex, I'd disconnect, like I was watching myself from up on the ceiling. My feelings of shame, guilt, and disgust persisted. As I worked through the memories of my abuse, I began to understand why I had always felt ashamed about my body and any positive physical sensations and why I'd always believed that love meant allowing someone to fuck me.

I had only ever really felt a physical connection to a very tiny spot in my body, a place in the middle of my body, just below my sternum and above my belly button. This spot mostly felt like a tight little knot. In my mind, if I stayed small, I could stay safe. I knew that if I was going to survive, I would have to take the risk to begin connecting with my whole body. But my body felt like the enemy. It held negative sensations and reminders of how I had been hurt and betrayed. I wanted to heal, but as I healed, more memories surfaced, and I'd retreat into my tiny, safe belly spot. I felt trapped.

## Enter Yoga

As a little girl I practiced yoga with my mum, and it felt special because it was something that only we shared. She spent so much time helping others and doing yoga with her made me feel that I mattered and was special. This ended when I had to go to school, and after she died these good memories were buried by my grief.

I was reintroduced to yoga just as the memories of abuse surfaced. I remembered how much I loved doing yoga with my mum but assumed my happy memories were all about spending time alone with her, not about the practice. I was skeptical because I was still using intense exercise to control my feelings and thoughts. Now that my truth had surfaced, I felt more desperate than ever to control and avoid my body. I finally knew why I was disconnected from my physical body, and the idea of consciously connecting to it was terrifying. But I knew my only way forward was to face myself, so I agreed to attend a class. To my utter amazement, during that first class I experienced a revelation. My body actually felt good, and I realized I had found what I had been searching for all my life: through yoga I might one day feel at home in my own skin. I was instantly hooked, but this time on something positive.

Change does not come easily, and for the first few years I tried to force my body into poses, not yet ready to listen to it. I still wanted to be in control. I liked the physical challenge and believed that through yoga I could *force* my body to be my ally. I had no idea what yoga was really about yet. As I began to feel connected to my physical body, new painful memories would surface, and I continued to struggle. Yoga became my salvation and my burden. And I continued to use food to help manage my emotions, to hide my secrets.

In 1999 I travelled to India and trained as a yoga instructor. There I learned that the recovery program I was living was actually ancient yogic wisdom and that the two paths I was travelling were one. I learned that the physical practice was only a very small part of yoga and that I had been using a sacred practice to attempt to control my enemy, my body. It was in India that I finally gave up the fight and began to make friends with my body.

## Ready to Hear the Message

In 2001, I was introduced to Bryan Kest, the founder of Santa Monica Power Yoga and Meditation. I was skeptical but agreed to attend a weekend workshop with him. I am grateful that I was willing to be open-minded about this guy because he was not like anyone I had met before. Bryan encouraged me to listen to my own body, to let my body be my yoga teacher. I know this message is not unique to him, but Bryan came into my life when I was finally ready to hear it. I learned that how I feel is more important than how I look and that the physical poses are merely opportunities to practice being fully present—body, mind, and spirit.

Very slowly I began to make friends with my body as I developed my own practice and actually began to look forward to exploring new parts of my body. I felt as if I was growing up physically, like I was beginning to fill up all the little nooks and crannies of my body. I no longer needed to stay safe in my tiny belly. I quit running and gave away my scale. I have not checked my weight in years, now trusting how my body feels rather than some arbitrary number.

Today I can sit quietly and experience my thoughts and feelings without judgment or reaction. Yoga's teachings allowed me to begin to accept myself as I am, not as I think I am supposed to be and to connect with my entire body in a safe, gentle, and loving way. Today I know I am perfect as I am, that there is no goal I need to attain. I have found the freedom to be me.

In the ancient yogic tradition, I now pass Bryan's teachings on to my own students, instructing in a variety of community and studio settings. I work at an addiction recovery home, and we include yoga as part of our programming. In collaboration with the center, I offer donation-based yoga classes open to the community. The donations collected support the residents of the center, who often come to us with little or nothing. I am honored to have the opportunity to pass on what has been given to me.

Does this mean I am comfortable in my own skin now? Most of the time, yes. Recovery is a journey, and I have learned that it is the most difficult experiences that offer me the biggest opportunities to grow. Sometimes I still burst into tears in the middle of a practice as my body allows me to connect with new memories. But sometimes I stop in my tracks, realizing I feel happy, joyous, and free. At these times I thank the people who helped me along the way, who loved me when I could not love myself. Until I came to yoga, I felt that my body was my enemy. Today I know my body is my most sacred partner and I love her, fiercely.

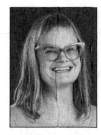

Jan Adams has been advocating and working in the fields of addiction, harm reduction, HIV/AIDS, and HCV since 1991. She has been instructing yoga since 1999 and is the owner of Northern Raven Yoga, a donation-based program. Jan is a grateful stepmum and granny. She lives in Thunder Bay, Canada, with her partner, Patrick, and their feline companions in a small, environmentally friendly home. Visit her at https://www.northernravenyoga.com/home. Follow her on Instagram at @kittygi62.

Author photo by Chondon Photography.

# RISE AND ALIGN: EMPOWERMENT AND CONNECTION AFTER TRAUMA AND ADDICTION

*Nicole Lang*

I was six years sober, and in the fifth year of my college career, when I finally and fully understood that I was a traumatized woman. It was fall and I was in a discussion for a class at Berkeley called the Anthropology of Violence and Trauma. We began the discussion reading from a book that Judith Herman, a psychiatrist who works with veterans and women who have experienced sexual violence, had written, which ended with this passage: "Traumatic events overwhelm the ordinary systems of care that give people a sense of control, connection, and meaning ... [They] are extraordinary, not because they occur rarely, but rather because they overwhelm the ordinary human adaptations to life."[1]

I had an almost out-of-body experience as we read those words. In that moment, a wave of memory and emotion washed over me, and sitting there at the start of term in a prestigious academic setting, it was

1. Judith Lewis Herman, *Trauma and Recovery: The Aftermath of Violence—From Domestic Abuse to Political Terror* (New York: Basic Books, 1992), 33.

as if I experienced all over again the trauma I thought I had put behind me. I now know I was having a post-traumatic stress response. I began to understand that my personal trauma was not something that could be judged or weighted by a person outside of myself, rather that trauma is an affliction of those who felt powerless and as if their essential selves had been overwhelmed by an outside force. In this one moment, sitting in that classroom, I knew that my trauma was real, that it ran deep into my past, that it had affected every aspect of my life, and that it was time to shed light on what that meant.

## Loss of Connection

I knew I was an alcoholic the first time I took a drink. There was nothing special about that day. I don't remember anything good or bad happening that led me to want to drink. I was twelve, it was after school, I had heard people talk about it, and I decided I wanted to get drunk. What I do remember is that as soon as I took a drink nothing mattered. The pain, the divorce, none of it affected me. After that first drink, I believed I had found the answer to life. I knew in my bones that drinking was for me. I had found "IT," and I didn't even know I was looking for it. That "IT" ended up being something outside of myself that could take over my senses and emotions with the first drink or hit. At that time in my life I wanted to be anyone but me, I didn't want to feel what I was feeling, and I was more than happy not to be responsible for any decisions.

It was no coincidence that my first drink came shortly after my parents divorced. The divorce was devastating to my entire family. It was destructive, fueled by anger and recrimination, and there seemed to be little thought of me and my sister, even though much of the fighting centered around who we would live with. And while the battles felt endless and without any hope of resolution, it seemed to us that neither of our parents were actually focused on taking care of us. I turned to drugs and alcohol; my sister turned inward, becoming quiet and shy.

Though alcohol remained my first love, I started smoking pot at thirteen, and what followed was a year of experimentation with hallucinogens, specifically LSD and mushrooms. I have memories of feeling depressed from a very early age, and the drugs and alcohol seemed to temporarily take it all away. I still don't know if the depression came because I was an alcoholic or if I was born with depression and it expressed itself in alcoholism. Either way, I do know that my depression and addiction went hand in hand. Drinking and using were the only coping skills I felt I had and the only ones I used. What I know now is that the depression was a result of trauma that took place when I was a young child, and the subsequent addiction was a new way for me to cope with that trauma. The interesting thing is, the more I used, the more trauma I incurred.

## Out-of-Body Experience

When I was fifteen, I began two life-altering relationships. The first was a seven-year relationship with an older man who I can see now was a sexual predator. He was five years my senior when we met. I started my relationship with him after the first time he raped me. At the time, I saw it as a sign of love and being wanted, as twisted as that may sound. The second was a five-year relationship with methamphetamine, introduced to me by that same man the first night we met. I barely got out of these relationships alive. It was in this seven-year period that most of my traumatic experiences occurred—either as a result of feeding my addiction to meth or my addiction to this man. I did whatever it took to maintain these relationships.

I dropped out of high school and moved out on my own. Well, I wasn't actually on my own, I had moved in with the man and whatever friends he had staying with him at any given time. I was a young teenage girl living in a house full of men in their twenties and thirties, some of whom cooked meth in the storage room, and most of whom viewed me as a sexual toy that could be used. I was in constant fear of what could happen to me at any given moment. Yet, somehow, I got used to the fear. Or maybe, now that I reflect on it, I was addicted to the fear and the attention. Having a possessive and volatile partner kept the harm from other dangerous men at bay, and I did enough harm to myself.

I now understand that I used my addiction as a way to disassociate from my body, and when I didn't have drugs or alcohol, I would use pain.

Cutting and suicide attempts were common methods for me to ease the pain. To be honest, they were common even when drugs and alcohol were part of the equation. There were countless occasions where, after a night of blacking out, I would come to with bandages on my wrists and questions about where I had ended up and how the cuts had gotten there. I didn't view myself, my body, or my life as having worth or value. Looking back now, it's clear I didn't know how to manage emotional pain. I did not allow myself to experience sadness, grief, or despair. I saw emotion and vulnerability as weakness, and I had to tell myself and believe that I was not weak. I was lost and scared and unable to connect with any kind of vulnerability. So I numbed myself to all of it and directed my pain outward. It was all I knew.

While others my age were gaining social skills learned from friends and teachers and mentors at high school, I was learning my social skills from addicts and drug dealers and from people whose only interest in me had to do with getting their next hit or getting access to my body. At this age, this was my world. These were my people, and it was all that I knew. None of us had any hope or goals other than staying loaded and not getting caught by the cops. Any friends I had were long gone or at arm's length. They couldn't stand to watch what I was doing to myself, or they could no longer trust me in their homes, or both.

By the time I turned eighteen, I was a criminal and an addict. My family did the best they could with what they had to manage and help me. But I was volatile, determined, addicted, and stubborn. I know this was a very difficult time for my family, and we are all very grateful that I made it out alive. Most young women in that same position do not. I remember sharing my story when I was newly sober, and afterward a gentleman came up to me, and with a seriousness in his face, said, "You are one in a million. You are a miracle. Never forget that. And share with others like you what has kept you alive."

## Finding Practice

Despite my best efforts to drink and die by twenty-five, with the help of a DUI, a judge, a probation officer, and a treatment counselor, I found myself getting sober at the age of twenty-one. I ended up finding real, solid sobriety in the meeting rooms of 12-step groups. It took time for the idea of sobriety to stick. When you can't imagine living in a world without drinking and using, it doesn't make sense for someone to ask you not to. Not only did it sound boring to my twenty-one-year-old self, it also sounded utterly terrifying. It also meant that I would have to stop numbing. I had been numbing myself for ten years, and I didn't know what to do when I started feeling again. That is what the 12-step groups started to help me with. They gave me principles to live by and a life to live for, but the program lacked the tools to help me get reconnected to my internal world. They helped me right my wrongs and make amends, but they didn't teach me how to connect with my body.

That is where yoga saved my life. I took my first yoga class when I was six months sober. At first, yoga was nothing more than physical exercise. The years of hard drugs and alcohol had taken their toll on my body. I had never been physically active or had any interest in health and wellness, didn't know how to sit still, be quiet, or listen to the "voice within." At the time, this all seemed ridiculous to me. As a way to deflect, I was loud and outspoken. I couldn't stop moving; I fidgeted all the time. Initially, the practices that worked best for me were fast-paced and physically demanding and allowed me to exhaust my body in order to exhaust my mind. Power practices allowed me to lie exhausted in savasana for a few short minutes without the desire to instantly get up off the mat. And even that took time. Yoga was made accessible to me through strong practices, which kept me interested and, most importantly, showed me a new way of connecting to my body.

I would tag along with friends who had YMCA memberships, and eventually I found a Rodney Yee yoga DVD on a discount store shelf that I would use for a home practice. For the majority of my yoga journey, I couldn't afford to practice at studios, buy a gym membership, or even pay for the cheapest classes in town. I would write down postures and sequences from classes I would take and make them my own. Yoga became so important to my daily routine that I sought it out where I could and did what I had to do to make it happen. The relationship I gained with my practice and my mat began to transform my inner landscape.

After a few years, the four corners of my yoga mat became boundaries to a sacred space that I could take with me anywhere. I was empowered and in control of everything within the edges of the mat. I was listening to and in control of my body for the first time in my life.

## Finding Connection

During the first few years of my sobriety, I decided to go back to school. Having earned my GED while I was still drinking in order to work full time, I started taking classes at the local community college. The longer I worked on my sobriety, and the more I practiced yoga, I found that I started to thrive in my life, particularly in school.

Soon after returning to school, I packed everything I owned into the back of my car one summer and moved to California. I had a bed in the back of my car, a makeshift kitchen, and my yoga mat. I would roll out my mat first thing in the morning in the mountains of Northern California. I'd watch surfers in Pismo Beach from my mat at 5 a.m. I found solace, comfort, and empowerment in my practice and took it with me wherever I would go. Eventually, I moved into a sober-living house in Santa Barbara and started classes at the city college.

To my great surprise, I was accepted to UC Berkeley with a full scholarship in 2012. I moved to Berkeley and found a donation-based yoga studio called Yoga to the People. This was the first time I practiced yoga with a teacher, in person, where I could ask questions and get guidance, and it allowed me to deepen my practice in ways I never imagined. It's also where I learned to cry on my mat. I cried during half pigeon and savasana for the two years I practiced at the studio. I was accessing emotions that had been physically lodged in my body since I was a young child. I still didn't understand what was happening to me at the time, but I could feel something was shifting. My home practice became a devotion and ritual to myself rather than just a physical exercise, and I started to not just listen to my muscles and joints but to hear what my whole body was saying.

Which brings me back to that moment in the violence and trauma class. While I originally focused my studies on archaeology, it was the classes on trauma and pain, the classes on communities of healing, that spoke to me. I think these classes helped me to understand intellectually what I had been feeling in my practice: that the work I was doing on my mat to develop safety and comfort allowed me to access the traumas that were being held in my hips, my legs, my shoulders, and in my heart.

The idea that one would have the right to control their own body is probably obvious to many, but this was something that I was never taught as a young woman. During the most important stages of social development, I had been raped and abused by others and controlled by substances, and what I learned—what was seared into my subconscious—was the exact opposite of control of my body. With the help of 12-step programs, years of work with therapists, and my yoga practice, I was on a path of recovery and healing. A path I still walk today. As a thirty-four-year-old mother, wife, and yoga instructor, I still struggle with depression, still can't escape entirely the memories and feelings of my trauma, and yet I keep coming back to that sacred space between the four corners of my yoga mat, and it always opens ways inside of me that need healing and attention. And now that I can get still enough and quiet enough to listen, I can find what I need to continue my journey of healing.

## A Call to Serve

I believe what the gentleman from the 12-step program told me many years ago is true. It is a miracle that I survived, and I have a responsibility to share with others what has helped me heal. I decided to become a yoga instructor and to seek out training in trauma-sensitive practices in order to guide and to share what I have experienced and learned with others like me, and with others whose experiences are different than mine, but who have the shared experience of trauma.

It took me six years to realize just how powerful my yoga practice was in my life, six years to understand the connection between yoga and trauma, and six years to be able to actively participate in my healing through my yoga practice. If I can share my experiences, knowledge, and the research I've done, share with my students what I've learned from the mistakes I've made, I hope maybe to empower them so they can make their journeys in less time. It is my passion to offer trauma-sensitive, affordable, and donation-based accessible yoga practices to young women, at-risk youth, and people in underserved communities. I would not trade a moment of my experience because it has made me the woman I am today, but I would not wish my experiences on anyone else. While trauma took away my sense of control, connection, and meaning, my yoga practice has given all those back to me and so much more. I am grateful to the light that yoga shined on all the dark shadows with me, that it lights my path and the paths of others who walk beside me toward love, compassion, and healing. Namaste.

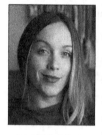

Nicole Lang is a trauma-informed certified yoga teacher, activist, speaker, and podcaster. In 2016, she created Rise & Align, a platform offering free and donation-based yoga for adolescents, young adults, individuals in recovery, and communities that have experienced trauma. She is currently working toward her MA in counseling psychology at Pacifica Graduate Institute. Learn more at www.riseandalign.com.

# ASANA, SELF-MORTIFICATION, AND THE MYTH OF THE HARDWORKING YOGI

## Colin Hall

As with smoking, drinking, food, and sex, it is possible to develop an unhealthy relationship with yoga postures. The ritual of a modern postural yoga class can be a rejuvenating and rewarding part of your day. But it can also become associated with some compulsive and obsessive behaviors.

I want to explore some of the deeper roots of addictive and obsessive behavior in yoga. I have noticed a few trends and issues that may shine some much-needed light. First, people spending too much time obsessing over their bodies is not a modern or recent development in yoga. There is a temptation to chalk up such behavior to social media; however, the history indicates otherwise. Second, there is an element of what sociologist Max Weber called the Protestant work ethic at play, which may be exacerbating an already unfortunate situation. Simply put, we have associated being a good person with being a hardworking person, and this may have dangerous consequences for yogis for whom *asana* (physical practice) is their primary practice. Finally, the ascetic and self-mortifying practices common to medieval hatha yogis have found their way into a modern practice that often advertises itself as a therapeutic or healing modality. These ascetic practices are not intended as a form of therapy but as a means to a kind of embodied spiritual freedom. The confusion between medieval metaphysical practices and modern therapeutic practices has serious consequences for contemporary yoga practitioners.

I do not mean to suggest that either medieval or modern yogis have a problem or that anybody is doing something wrong. As another famous sociologist, Emile Durkheim, would have said, these are social facts. It is not for me to judge whether or not yogis should put themselves through self-mortifying practices. Clearly addiction and compulsion both have terrible personal and social costs, but I want to be very clear that not all addictions should be treated equally. It is possible to, in the words of my yoga teacher, David McAmmond, "trade up" our addictions from less to more healthy ones.

An alcoholic who starts drinking coffee to help kick alcohol still has an addiction. But it is a better addiction. Similarly, somebody dealing with a substance addiction or other forms of obsessive-compulsive behaviors who develops a yoga addiction should not be judged. They should be commended. That was an excellent trade.

There are, however, some serious problems associated with yoga addiction and yoga compulsion that we can discuss without casting judgment on people who are just trying to improve their lives. By getting more clarity about the potential dangers of excessive yoga practice, we may be able to minimize the risks posed to those of us with compulsive or addictive yoga behaviors.

Perhaps even more interesting still is the possibility that we might, along the way, shine a light on a harmful relationship with our bodies that lurks quietly in the corners of yoga studios and gyms around the world. Veiled by vague notions like wellness, self-loathing is much more common among yoga practitioners and teachers than we might imagine.

## The Quest for Yoga Realness

When I started teaching yoga in the early 2000s, I was not what you would call a typical yogi. Years of speedskating left my hamstrings feeling like piano wire. I was a singer in a punk band and was used to screaming into a microphone rather than speaking in hushed tones to near-sleeping students on yoga mats.

Which meant I often felt like I did not fit in. I regularly found myself in rooms full of beautiful people wearing coordinated outfits and executing postures with apparent ease while I was awkwardly trying to stop quivering while wearing Calvin Klein pajamas. When I went into yoga workshops, I felt like a teenager trying to fit in with a bunch of adults at a cocktail party. Completely out of place.

So I tried to make myself look the part. I couldn't grow a decent beard, and I didn't want to have to take care of long hair. I didn't have any mala beads, tattoos of Indian deities, or abdominal muscles to flex. All I had were the postures. I did my best to make my postures look like the photos I saw in the books. The postures of David Swenson, B. K. S. Iyengar, and Erich Schiffmann became like idealized shapes for me that I attempted to mimic.

It didn't work very well. In a few years of daily rigorous asana practice, I never really progressed all that far. I did manage to hurt my back a number of times. I tore my right hamstring twice. I demonstrated postures only on my "good side" because I wanted to impress my students. I caused a significant asymmetry in my legs, which I believe continues to inspire the occasional SI joint flare-up today.

When I started yoga, I was inflexible and it showed. After a few years, I was still inflexible, but I was able to make people believe that I could do all the poses. I practiced long and hard, but not to make my body healthier. I practiced so that I could demonstrate my membership in club yoga. Because I correlated my asana practice with approval and acceptance in the "yoga scene," I was set up for an unhealthy relationship with the postures.

## The History of Self-Mortification in Yoga

Hatha yoga (what I'll just refer to as "yoga" here on out) is roughly one thousand years old and started with Buddhist and Shaiva (Shiva-worshipping) Tantric sects who took an unorthodox view of *moksha*, or liberation. In classical yoga, moksha is the release of the self from the bonds of the body. Your consciousness is untethered from the constantly changing world of materiality, and you experience yourself as a subject without an object. It is a state of oneness in which there is no body, no ego, no thoughts, imagination, memory, or identity.

The tantrics took an entirely different view of liberation. They believe in liberation in this world, not the next. Liberation in the body. It was referred to as *jiva mukti*, or embodied freedom. Because there is no distinction between the self and the world, because everything is made from the same material, because both consciousness and the body have a common source, then there is no need to escape the body in order to experience freedom. This was the beginning of hatha yoga.

Hatha yogis developed a system of practices designed to purify the physical body. It needed to be cleansed in order to be an effective vehicle or host for an embodied form of liberation. These practices take a number of different forms. Some of them are attempts to physically cleanse the body (*kriyas*) while others are an attempt to overcome weakness and establish the dominance of the will over the inclinations of the physical body. I should add that many of the bandhas (subtle energy locks), mudras (gestures—similar to asanas), and kriyas (cleansing techniques) of medieval hatha yoga were less about purification and more about creating upward, rather than downward, flow of energy in the body.

Energy going down is bad. Energy going up is good.

The kriyas were consciously excluded from the practices exported from India in the twentieth century that became what we know as modern postural yoga. This was an intentional omission by yoga icons like Vivekananda who believed, rightly, that American and European sensibilities would be offended by practices like *vaman dhauti* where you drink water and induce vomiting to cleanse the stomach.

Other kriyas involved more intense and dramatic actions. For example, the *Hatha Yoga Pradipika* recommends a practice called *khechari mudra* in which the lingual frenulum (the skin that connects your tongue to the bottom of your mouth) is severed and the tongue is stretched over the course of months in order to be capable of putting the tongue behind the soft palate and up into the nasal cavity.[2]

And to think, I was feeling stressed about trying to hold headstand. Modern yogis have it easy.

While I never had to sever part of my tongue, it seems some of these ancient asceticisms did not remain in medieval history but found their way into modern practice. The three bandhas practiced in Ashtanga vinyasa, hanging upside down, exposure to heat, some Kundalini breathing exercises, and putting your leg behind your head are all examples of hatha yoga asceticism that is practiced by modern yogis. All of these things are potentially dangerous actions that, performed obsessively or compulsively, could result in injury or disorder.

## Yoga and the Protestant Work Ethic

I don't have time for a detailed discussion of Max Weber's classic book *The Protestant Ethic and the Spirit of Capitalism*. It's a good read though. Don't let the very academic-sounding title put you off. The basic idea is that Protestants, and Calvinists in particular, believed in predestination. Which means God has already chosen which of us will be saved and go to heaven and which of us are basically destined for an afterlife in hell. This led to social anxiety because Protestants had no way of knowing who was who. Worldly success, like a booming business, came to be seen as a kind of indicator for who had God's grace. The more you buckled down, saved your pennies, reinvested in your business rather than spending on things you enjoy, and neglected holidays and rest, the more your business would thrive, and you could rest assured that you must be one of the elect.[3]

This ethic is at work today in what is called "performative wellness." The better shape you are in, the more chiseled your abs, the healthier your meals, the less cluttered your home, are all indicators of grace. You must be destined for success. So people knock themselves out in an

2. Svatmarama, *The Hatha Yoga Pradipika*, trans. Brian Dana Akers (New Delhi, India: New Age Books, 2002), 59–61.

3. Weber, Max, *The Protestant Ethic and the Spirit of Capitalism*, trans. Stephen Kalberg (Abingdon, Oxon: Routledge, 2013).

effort to demonstrate how healthy they are. It is simultaneously a signal to your community that you are one of the chosen and, at the same time, a way to reassure yourself that your life has meaning and purpose.

This was encapsulated by the now disgraced guru of Ashtanga vinyasa yoga Pattabhi Jois when he said, "Anyone can practice. Young man can practice. Old man can practice. Very old man can practice. Man who is sick, he can practice. Man who doesn't have strength can practice. Except lazy people; lazy people can't practice yoga."[4]

Only the lazy can't do yoga. What does that say about people who just don't have the time, energy, or money to commit to a regular yoga practice? The people who are injured and need to rest? The people who want to spend time with their family instead of at the yoga studio? According to Jois, those people are lazy and, as a result, not yogis.

A hard-headed commitment to yoga practice is often viewed as a mark of good character. It means you take your practice seriously and is often associated with spiritual accomplishment. Nearly every yoga teacher is almost obliged to talk about how hard they worked to achieve the postures they now demonstrate with ease.

How often have you heard a yoga teacher who was an ex-dancer or gymnast say something like, "These poses are super easy compared to the contortions required of me when I was dancing"? How often do you hear yoga teachers saying they are just naturally flexible and so were able to do advanced postures nearly effortlessly from the first few classes they took? Yoga teachers with natural flexibility are rarely open and honest about it. More often than not they will make it seem like their flexibility came as a result of years of hard work and commitment.

Self-sacrifice is the measure of success. Success in yoga without some kind of personal hardship is seen as a shortcut or somehow not authentic or "real enough."

4. YJ Editors, "Practice and All is Coming," YogaJournal.com, Cruz Bay Publishing, updated April 12, 2017, https://www.yogajournal.com/yoga-101/practice-and -all-is-coming-2; "Building a Community Through the Practice of Ashtanga Yoga," Ashtanga Yoga, n.d., https://www.ashtangayoga302.com.

## Asana Addiction

Yogis can develop an unhealthy relationship to asana practice in a number of different ways. An asana addiction develops when the pleasurable sensations associated with stretching become something that you need to feel regularly. Like opiates, an increase in dosage is required in order to create the same level of stimulation. Think about the first time you really stretched out your hamstrings. Especially how they felt immediately after the pose. It is an electrically charged bliss. But after five to ten years, it just feels like another hamstring stretch. Still nice, but not electric bliss.

I think of this like the yoga version of chasing the dragon. We want that same feeling but need bigger and more intense postures in order to re-create it. The same thing can happen with affirmation and approval. The first time you do an arm balance you might get all kinds of applause and adulation. Everybody is so happy for you. You did it! But what about after five to ten years of arm balances? Now nobody cares about a simple little arm balance. If it isn't balancing on one arm at the edge of a cliff, does it even count?

That is addiction. Yoga produces a physical or emotional pleasure that results in powerful cravings. These cravings make asana-addicted yogis start ignoring family, work, injuries, and the rest of the world, generally speaking, so that they can focus on chasing more pleasure.

An obsessive relationship with asana practice is different from asana addiction. It involves little to no pleasure. It was, I imagine, much more common for medieval hatha yogis who most likely did not enjoy hanging upside down while swinging through a fire (yes, that is a thing). Their practice was not a source of pleasure but rather a kind of requirement arising from their identity as a yogi.

If you are seriously committed to your asana practice, but everything else in your life is ticking along just fine, you are probably not compulsive and should not stress over it. But if your practice is regularly resulting in injuries, if anti-inflammatories are required in order for you to practice, or if you find that the rest of your life is chaotic and yoga practice feels like the only reprieve from an otherwise unpleasant life, you may be developing an unhealthy relationship to your asana practice.

## Some Suggestions

There is a power to ritual action that is comforting in times of distress. When anxiety arises, we all have ritual movements and actions that we use to make us feel better. I have a funny habit of spinning my wedding ring on my finger. It has no significance or special meaning other than giving me something to do with my hands, which I find comforting. When these ritual actions cease to bring you any kind of comfort, it is time to start experimenting with new rituals and actions.

Maybe you always start your yoga practice with a seated meditation and a breathing exercise. If that is working for you there is no reason to change it. But if you find that your practice is no longer creating the same feelings of comfort and reassurance that it once did, you may need to change it up. Do not get stuck in yoga routines that start feeling … well … routine.

Yogis with an asana addiction may want to try stopping asana practice altogether for a short while. Notice if you tend to be angry or irritable if you miss your asana practice. Notice if you are no longer engaging in many social or leisure activities that are not asana related. These are symptoms of asana addiction and could be leading you toward mistreating, neglecting, or abusing your own body in an effort to continue your asana practice.

Find new ways to practice. Meditation and pranayama are wonderful alternatives to asana practice. Prayer, mantra, contemplation, journaling, reflection, volunteering, and reading are all ways of practicing yoga without asana. Giving up asana practice is not giving up yoga. Not even close.

It is possible to imagine that the postures we practice in asana classes are somehow sacred. We imagine asana practice as an integrated piece of a sacred whole called yoga. The truth is that most of the asana being practiced today is less than one hundred years old. Yes, people have been practicing postures for thousands of years. But they have not been moving through choreographed flows featuring creative transitions, unique modifications, and honed scripts designed to entertain and inspire. The yoga we are practicing today is not ancient nor is it more sacred than going for a walk, working in your garden, or playing with your children.

No need to be dramatic about it. You are not breaking up with asana practice for life. This isn't Romeo and Juliet. In a couple months, or even a couple years, maybe you will have time and space to reflect on the role of asana practice in your life. What does it really accomplish for you? Why do you practice it? If you do not have a good answer to those questions, maybe now is the time for a little break.

## References

Mallinson, James, and Mark Singleton, ed. and trans. *Roots of Yoga*. London: Penguin Books, 2017.

White, David Gordon, ed. *Yoga in Practice*. Princeton, NJ: Princeton University Press, 2012.

Samuel, Geoffrey. *The Origins of Yoga and Tantra: Indic Religions to the Thirteenth Century*. New York: Cambridge University Press, 2008.

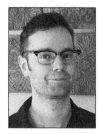

Colin Hall is a lecturer in religious studies and kinesiology at the University of Regina and has been teaching and studying yoga for over twenty years. He's the co-director of Bodhi Tree Yoga, where he and his wife, Sarah, have been building a thriving yoga community in the small prairie city of Regina, Saskatchewan. Colin started practicing in the late 1990s and continues to learn from his original teacher, David McAmmond. Learn more at www.bodhitreeyoga.com.

# UPRISING

*Jill Weiss Ippolito*

## Bikram Yoga Disclaimer

I've been asked to write a disclaimer about Bikram Yoga because this book and my work is about healing trauma. Many people are aware of several lawsuits against Bikram Choudhury and BY. I'm not the most outspoken on either subjects other than how the yoga practice set me on my path to healing trauma. UpRising Yoga started when I was working at the World Headquarters of Bikram Yoga. My time and experience with the BY community has been both loving and supportive as well as volatile, and ultimately a catalyst toward healing my own personal trauma.

---

"$10 for 10 days of hot yoga" the sign said at Silverlake BY. It was 2001. Nearby I was living in a Section 8 apartment in Silverlake, and fresh out of an institution due to struggles with substance abuse. My probation officer insisted that I follow the court conditions and seek sobriety and employment.

My first yoga class was torturous and painful, but the worst part about it was facing myself in the mirror.

Extremely frail, underweight, covered in bruises, my eyes looked dark and haunted. I had no idea who I was. My beliefs were distorted, causing me to think I was disgusting, overweight, and ugly. Such punishing and crippling thoughts. Often I stayed home with panic attacks, depression, and severe anxiety.

Detoxing from heroin use was easier than grasping a new way of living and forming healthy, life-supporting habits. Turns out the one that saved my life was yoga. Yet as much as I hated the entire ninety minutes of yoga (it was so hot I thought I was going to die!), practicing with people who were so focused and in sync to the poses, I became inspired. The instructor was encouraging and uplifting, offering suggestions I felt I could try. And the poses felt really good! And eventually, the heat did too. The cool air hit my face when I left that very first yoga class and it felt fresh on my skin as if a new wind of life was breezing by. I liked being alive for the first time.

From that moment on I decided that I needed more of it. Perhaps like addiction, I craved this intimate interaction with myself. Postures were cleansing, and with a familiar routine I started getting better at them relatively quickly, which helped me to soften the cruel thoughts about what I saw in the mirror. It would take years for me to truly connect and journey on toward self-love, but the more I went back to yoga, the easier it got and the better I felt.

When ten days were up and the shock of paying for a class membership sunk in, I walked up to the front desk ready to explode.

"I was tricked by your ad! I can't afford to pay twenty dollars a class and now I don't know what to do, I need to keep coming here!" I wailed at the smiling woman.

She asked, "Do you want to work here? We offer *seva*, a work trade karma yoga program where you work here in exchange for your yoga classes."

Hesitant but desperate I asked what I would be doing, and she said cleaning up the studio, vacuuming, cleaning the bathroom, restocking towels, wiping down the mats, whatever was needed. There was a condition I needed to follow and that was I had to agree to come to class three times a week. I agreed.

The instructors looked happy, as if they liked their lives. Soon I would get to know them. Once I asked one of the teachers how I was supposed to keep this up when I felt tired or strained; how could I continue on? She said all you have to do is *show up*. That showing up is the hardest part, and once you have made it to class it didn't matter what you did as far as postures went. If I did nothing but lie down on the mat in the back row, then that was my yoga for the day. My practice didn't have to look like anything. I only had to show up and listen to my body. Listen for the wisdom that emanates from within, listen to your body. I could do that, I thought, and felt entirely empowered. This phrase still helps me get to class today.

I held on to the notion that maybe I, too, could become a yoga instructor someday. I bought the book in the lobby and started asking a lot of questions. I even asked about what to eat, I had no idea.

But after practicing regularly for over a year, I couldn't continue thanks to my rigid and aggressive perfectionism with myself in the studio mirror. (Unlike many other types of studios, hot yoga studios have mirrors.) I was a fit model and a bit obsessed with my size. And if I fell out of a pose, I cussed out loud! I was a super thin, hungry, and angry lady. I looked like a sharp, angular little boy and wanted to be softer in body and essence. I decided to quit yoga and sit on a beach eating until I got curvy, feminine hips.

In reality, I took a year away from hot yoga and tried practicing several other styles before I went back. Once I saw my shape in the mirror again, I was so out of alignment it worried me. I decided right then to sign up for teacher training, not necessarily to teach, but to understand how I could use yoga to address my injuries. I put the training on my credit card and off I went.

## Becoming a Yoga Instructor

In 2006, I received my certification to teach hot yoga.

Giving back what had been freely given to me meant the world. It was a miracle to go from a miserable existence of struggle to teach two to four ninety-minute yoga classes a day, running from yoga studio to studio and actually earning enough rent money to scrape by. I loved carrying the message that yoga saved my life. This gave me a purpose and a community to embrace. I was passionate about letting people know that if I could do it anyone could!

Quickly, life improved and I was able to move out of my single studio, get a dog, and keep myself afloat teaching yoga. Eventually, though, the hustle of yoga classes and low wages took its toll. And over time, I became frustrated by how much wealth, youth, and beauty were valued in contemporary yoga culture. Still, yoga was it for me and I clung to it.

I craved more meaning in my world, and I was yearning to be of service. I wanted to share yoga with those who were not able to get to a yoga class, especially incarcerated youth. One thing that had inhibited me in the beginning was how much a yoga class cost, and I wondered how I could make yoga more affordable and accessible.

Along with a few other teachers, I started teaching yoga in juvenile hall. We went in as a group and over time I applied for a nonprofit and came up with the name UpRising Yoga.

Teaching yoga in juvenile hall was a window to my own youth: into the young angst, misery, rebellion, mischievousness, neglect, fear, and loneliness that led to my self-destructive behavior. I saw myself in the kids: hungry for love, acceptance, and safety. My household had been extremely erratic and violent, and I was very unsupervised. I knew that yoga gave me a reliance on myself, a foundation, and ultimately autonomy, and I wanted to pass this along to them.

I tried for a while to teach hot yoga in juvenile hall, but we weren't able to provide heat and mirrors. This led me to take teacher trainings in other styles of yoga, which gave me more of a variety to choose from when creating posture sequences. We introduced many types of yoga and included meditation and mindfulness. Because juvenile hall is transitional, oftentimes we only saw a student once, so I wanted to make sure that in every class we taught a life skill, a tool that could be used to foster resilience, such as breathing to calm down during court and other stressful times. One young woman in juvenile hall told me that she practiced breathing with her judge during her court case.

## The Present and the Future

Eight years have gone by now, and I have developed curriculums and teach trauma-informed yoga trainings worldwide.

UpRising Yoga now offers free weekly community yoga classes as well as gang prevention and aftercare programs all over Los Angeles. We have taught in schools, parks, youth camps, hospitals, institutions, group homes, and on skid row. Recently we taught one hundred students at a teen grief camp, which was a beautiful experience.

My recovery from addiction is linked to yoga, and my intention is to spread the UpRising Yoga model worldwide to bring together those doing this work, measure outcomes, and see more impact. My mission to ensure that yoga is seen as a healing modality and effective tool for those incarcerated is coming true, and my passion to make yoga affordable and accessible for marginalized communities continues to drive me.

I am always reminded that while everyone may need yoga healing across the globe, oftentimes the need is closer to home than imagined. Recently, our local grocery store had a hostage situation: a shooting that left the store manager dead and our town in shock and grief. I called a recovery house and asked if they would host a trauma-informed yoga class for the community to gather and heal together. It was an incredible class and a memorial for the victim. One of the survivors said that she felt safe and had received comfort from our class. Several days later, it dawned on me that is how UpRising Yoga started. I heard a need and leaped to offer what skills I had. It shows that we all can reach out and offer whatever we can in order to help ease the suffering of another. I'm grateful to pass this message along and to inspire others to do the same.

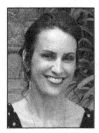 Jill Weiss Ippolito is a yoga educator and consultant, activist, public speaker, writer, and founder of the nonprofit UpRising Yoga, which offers yoga and life skills classes to underserved populations and communities. With Yoga for Healing Trauma, an international trauma-informed training program, Jill

educates numerous service providers, yoga instructors, childcare providers, educators, mental health professionals, and advocates for the reformation of prison and probation culture through yoga. Learn more at www.uprisingyoga.org.

Author photo by Alicia Bailey.

# SOBER LIVING, SEX, AND SURRENDER: WHAT YOGA TAUGHT ME

## David Holzer

I was forty-seven when I began practicing yoga. Lali, the love of my life up until then, had died three years previously in February 2005. In October 2008, after a spiritual retreat had somehow switched off my desire to drink, I got sober. Although it felt like tempting fate to say so, I'd gone sideways into a world where drink was for everyone else, not me. I was relieved.

For over thirty years, until it became a job that hurt, drinking had made the world go away, given me joy and illumination, and sent me off on mad adventures I would never regret. Even if some, like the time I ended up in an alley with two young guys waving knives at me or when I fell down a flight of stone stairs and almost broke my neck, now made me shudder.

At the time I began my life in yoga, the elation I'd felt at still being alive, free from cirrhosis and type 2 diabetes, and HIV negative had worn off. Without booze, I was living kind of how I assumed other people did. I had to adjust to a life without dramatic highs or lows. I had begun to grieve without an escape route.

The problem was that, although getting sober had saved my life, I didn't know how to live without booze. Getting out of my head had been part of my routine. Being a drinker had been fundamental to my idea of myself.

## Beginning with Kundalini Yoga

My journey into yoga began with Kundalini yoga. I wandered into a room in a spiritual center where I was living in Palma de Mallorca, the capital of the largest Spanish Balearic island, and saw a woman all in white wrapping a white turban around her head. She told me she was preparing to teach a Kundalini class and invited me to join. I ended up practicing with her for around a year. Although I loved the practice and it liberated inspiration for my writing to a remarkable extent, the best thing about Kundalini yoga for me was that it got me stoned.

I practiced Kundalini until I no longer needed to get out of my head so much. It helped me transition into sober living. After Kundalini, I went to hatha and then vinyasa flow. I took up vinyasa only because it was the main form of yoga offered by a studio in Palma that I'd fallen in love with.

When I began practicing at the studio, I was tattooed, bloated from years of drinking and a bad diet, poured with sweat, grunted, and practiced wearing black because I thought it made me look thinner. My face contorted in anger as I struggled with poses that everyone else seemed to float into effortlessly. The yoginis seemed wary around me. I've never thought of myself as scary, but perhaps I was. Also, even though I was no longer part of it, I was still locked into the mindset of the often cynical, nihilistic, and violent drinkers' world I'd escaped. I thought I kept it well-hidden, but the contempt I felt for the whole "no judgment" studio bubble—which I thought was fake—must have come off me in waves. I was a walking thundercloud.

Still, I went back to the studio again and again, practicing four times a week. I had become fascinated by yoga. Vinyasa was seriously challenging, and I would stumble out of each class exhausted and still pouring with sweat. But learning to occupy my body, concentrating on sending my breath to my left knee or right ankle—damaged by several drunken falls—was a revelation. Over time, I was able to practice without a knee or ankle support.

Yoga was also affecting my consciousness. Focusing on what was happening to my body in the moment enabled me to put my raw grief aside for a while. Being in the studio gave me purpose and helped me rise out of the profound sense of confusion I felt. At least when I was attempting a headstand, I knew precisely what I was doing, or attempting.

Although the effect wasn't as intense as with Kundalini yoga, practicing vinyasa also enabled me to access where words come from for me, to develop my powers of focus, concentration, and discipline.

After I'd made it home to my apartment and crawled into bed, sometimes after a morning class, my mind was sufficiently empty that I could sleep untroubled by agonizing dreams.

Put simply, yoga gave me something to do that wasn't drinking and a better me to aim for. I only realized how important this was years later when I studied addiction and recovery in more detail.

Those friends of mine who'd managed to quit booze and drugs but fell off the wagon always did so because they didn't have a good enough reason to stay sober. Yoga was my reason. As I came to appreciate the qualities of positivism, compassion, empathy, and lack of judgment, I tried to live up to them more and more.

## The Presence of Yoginis

The reasons I've given for why I fell in love with yoga and was driven to practice obsessively for the next seven years of my life are all true. But they don't tell the whole story.

From the very beginning, drink had given me the courage to try and initiate sexual encounters. On the first night we met, Lali and I had gotten wonderfully drunk and fallen into bed together. In the four years I carried on drinking after she died, I ended up in bed with women on several occasions, helped by booze.

When I stopped drinking, all that stopped. It was as if I'd been catapulted back into adolescence. I had evidence that I'd spent seven years with Lali—her photo was everywhere in our apartment, I couldn't bring myself to throw away her favorite pair of turquoise shorts, the packs of morphine patches from the last months of her life, or even remove her hairs from her hairbrush—but it was as if I'd never shared my life and bed with a living, breathing woman. Her death was the first thing in my life I'd been unable to run away from.

I didn't want another relationship, partly because Lali was still more real to me than the flesh and blood women I met, but also because I'd treated the women I'd been with after she'd died so badly. Despite feeling that getting involved with another woman would have been a betrayal to Lali, I naturally still wanted sex. At the same time, I couldn't imagine having sex again, not sober. I was deeply, profoundly confused. And it hurt.

What I didn't realize at the time was that it wasn't sex I was lacking. It was the balance provided by feminine energy that I'd had in my relationship with Lali. I eventually found that being in the fundamentally feminine space of the yoga studio I attended helped me heal and prepared me for reentering the world of relationships.

When I first saw a class practicing yoga, I thought the combination of grace, strength, and power was one of the most beautiful things I'd ever witnessed. I was moved to tears. A pure light of concentration and pleasure radiated from each student. Together, they shone. They were utterly in the moment of their practice. When they attempted a challenging asana, their courage was heroic.

As I evolved in my own practice, slowly my feeling that I was a tired old wolf among swans began to dissolve. I stopped sneering at the Rumi quote painted on the wall of the studio: "Out beyond ideas of wrongdoing and rightdoing, there is a field. I'll meet you there."[5] The yoga studio became that field for me.

When the only way you've seen someone is when they are practicing yoga, it can be easy to assume the whole of their life is the same. As I got to know them, I discovered that some of the people who I'd thought lived lives as graceful as their practice were dealing with trauma that was at the very least the equal of my own loss. A visiting yoga teacher had lost her husband and, I think, one of her sons in the 2004 Indian

---

5. Jala al-Din Rumi, *The Essential Rumi*, trans. Coleman Barks with John Moyne, A.J. Arberry, and Reynold Nicholson (New York: Castle Books, 1997).

Ocean tsunami and tried to drown herself in drink before finding yoga. Hearing her story and those of others humbled me, made me feel less alone, and gave me hope. If they could survive a mighty punch in the face from life, so could I. Self-pity was understandable but not useful. I would practice alternate nostril breathing until I stopped feeling sorry for myself.

It wasn't just being in the physical presence of these yoga practitioners that gave me comfort. The studio, its walls painted a cool cream color and its natural wood floors, became a sanctuary for me. I loved walking through the door and seeing the big bunch of pink, purple, or white lilies on the reception desk, the display cases filled with mala beads in orange, red, and turquoise hanging from hooks, the racks of yoga clothes adorned with giant, brilliantly colorful butterfly or unicorn designs one teacher brought back from Brazil. I loved smelling the sweet aromas of incense, herbal tea, deodorant, and honest perspiration. I learned to smile when teachers instructing a class would say, "Ladies and David."

I would arrive at the studio twenty minutes early and often be one of the last to leave.

## Learning to Surrender

I practiced at the studio three to four times a week and took part in workshops for the next seven years. In that time, several fellow yoga practitioners became good friends. For me, the studio remained a haven.

In that seven years, my grief settled into a sadness that slowly came to occupy less and less of my waking life. The moments when I would feel pain so raw my breath would catch and a single moaning sob would escape became fewer. I let go of much of my anger at the world, and the set of my mouth softened from its perpetual downward-turned scowl. Some of the hurt went out of my eyes. Surrendering to challenging yoga poses and accepting there were some things I'd simply never be able to do helped I'm sure.

Eventually, I accepted that my next relationship had to be entirely adult. I had to find the courage to risk everything. Perhaps finding the nerve to get into yoga poses I found scary had something to do with this. I'd like to think so. I became a little braver every day. It was a sensible courage. Because yoga had helped me manage my pain and I knew I could wait, I surrendered to time.

When the wonderful woman I'm with today chose me, I was amazed to find that I'd fallen completely in love with her without having to deny any of my feelings for and memories of Lali. I believe this is because of the way I'd learned to experience powerful emotion in my yoga practice, while also holding it up to the light. Yoga had made my sense of my interior space larger, which allowed the multitudinous feelings I contained to coexist. Finding sanctuary in the yoga studio surrounded by women gave me the space I needed to heal.

I'll always be grateful.

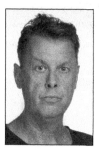

David Holzer is a professional writer and yogi. He began practicing around ten years ago. Since then, yoga has become an integral part of David's life and work. He teaches yoga for writers and writing for yogis.

Author photo by Fuji Foto Central.

# PART ONE: REFLECTION QUESTIONS

- What do you hear when you get still and quiet enough to listen?
- What is one truth your practice of yoga has revealed to you that has been difficult to accept?
- What patterns has your practice revealed that you want to shift or change?
- How has your practice supported you in changing your relationship with things that cause harm to your mind, body, and spirit?

—Michelle C. Johnson

# PART TWO

## *Healing and Thriving*

Each individual's healing journey from physical trauma and illness is unique. It can be unwise and unhealthy to compare our experiences to those of others (especially the fictional or glorified triumphs of a few). It can also be unwise or unhealthy to compare our present selves to past versions of ourselves. By dropping these comparisons and expectations, we increase the possibility of allowing ourselves to develop acceptance and compassion for where we're at in the present moment and where we're headed, as well as extend that same acceptance and compassion to the journeys others navigate.

As Jennifer Kreatsoulas bravely shares in "Revising the Terms of Eating Disorder Recovery," it's critical that we not only rethink the ways we think about "eating disorders," "mental illness," "healing," and "recovery" (which may include one or more relapses), we need to change the way we relate to and talk about them. There is much healing to gain and resilience to experience when we begin to consciously revise our language and reorient the ways in which we relate to the diagnoses and recovery journey.

Mary Higgs employed her curiosity over and over again to allow the accident that left her with a spinal cord injury teach her how to become more resilient and offer her wisdom to support and inspire the healing of others. Admittedly, the road wasn't easy and took years, but she continued to use her practices to shift her challenges into opportunities to grow her confidence, increase her courage, and expand her capacity to teach and serve others. None of it was expected; all of it was fuel for her healing.

In "From Pain to Empowerment," Sarah Garden shares the intimate and powerful details of her journey from her endometriosis diagnosis and the lack of agency she felt to reclaiming agency and control over her body, her healing, and her own health. Not only did Sarah learn how to feel empowered and dignified in her body again, she's also leading the way for others to do the same—in large part by utilizing yoga and mindfulness techniques. Not only can we redefine our relationships to our bodies and learn new ways to manage the pain we may experience, we can also redefine what healing and "health care" look like.

The first time Amanda Huggins remembers experiencing anxiety, she was fourteen years old. Something that she initially talked about as "that feeling" became a frequent and familiar experience over the years, one that she was finally able to identify and name. Yet despite that ability, not only did anxiety become part of her everyday life, guilt and shame for "having anxiety" were part of the package. Though yoga first left her feeling like she wanted to escape, eventually Amanda became able to meet her "triggers on the mat" and to explore her anxiety in a new way. She discovered that she could expand her self-awareness and heal through a variety of tools, some of which were prescribed by others and some that she uncovered through her own experience. In the end, in unexpected ways as a result of her yoga and mindfulness practice, she was able to move fully into purpose.

Sarah Harry ponders her ability to teach yoga after an accident left her with a shattered kneecap and the discovery that she had incurable osteoarthritis in "Will I Ever Teach Yoga Again?" For a well-known international yoga teacher, this is a sobering question to ask: a question that left Sarah in a state of deep grieving and loss (as well as incredible amounts of physical pain). Yet it was her years of continuous mental and physical practice that allowed her a new opportunity to experience and move past her anger and depression as well as her traumatic relationship to pain. With mindfulness and patience, Sarah has redefined not only her yoga practice and how she moves in her body but how she teaches and guides others to do the same.

# MEDITATION

## *I Am Healing, Whole, and Thriving*

For this practice please find an object that represents wholeness to you. If you cannot find an object then please write down the words "healing," "whole," and "thriving" on a piece of paper (creating a mantra card), and place your object or the mantra card near you for this meditation.

We will start with a breathing practice to quiet your mind.

Find a comfortable seat or, if you prefer, you can stand or lie down. Place your object next to you or near you.

To find a comfortable seat, you might want to elevate your hips by sitting on a cushion, pillow, or blanket.

Close your eyes or look at the ground in front of you and begin to breathe into your body. Start by taking deep breaths in and out. Begin to notice the expansion as you breathe in and the contraction or release with your exhale.

Now, continue to breathe.

Take deep belly breaths, inhaling and feeling the energy move up and exhaling, feeling the energy move down.

Sit for at least three minutes, breathing deeply into your belly.

Take a moment to be with yourself here, fully. Allow yourself to be here, to be present.

Bring your awareness to the object or mantra card and notice the energy it is offering to you.

If you would like, you can repeat the mantra three times:

"I am whole."

"I am healing."

"I am thriving."

Notice how you feel as you work with this mantra. You are whole, healing, and thriving.

Once you feel ready to move out of meditation, with each breath cycle bring your awareness back to deep belly breaths and the expansion and contraction and release. Return to the space by opening your eyes and take a moment to notice how you feel. Honor your feelings.

—Michelle C. Johnson

# REVISING THE TERMS OF EATING DISORDER RECOVERY

*Jennifer Kreatsoulas*

On Mother's Day of 2014, I went for a walk in Philadelphia's Wissa-hickon Valley Park with my husband and two daughters to celebrate the gift of motherhood and the blessing of my children. My then two-year-old daughter held her father's hand as I pushed our ten-month-old daughter in her stroller along the gravel path. Under the bright sun of early spring, runners, cyclists, dog walkers, and the occasional horse-back rider navigated around families like mine who were enjoying the holiday in this idyllic place.

From the outside, our family fit perfectly into this blissful scene. We smiled, laughed, and skipped rocks in the creek. The girls petted the dogs and fed the ducks. Between the beauty of the natural landscape and our togetherness, we appeared the epitome of familial happiness.

The truth: I was dying on the inside, and no matter how cheerful this scene appeared, I was too physically weak and mentally cloudy to fully experience any of it.

The stress of being a new mother, coupled with sleep deprivation, postpartum depression, and the absence of self-care had resulted in a severe relapse of anorexia nervosa. Now, in my late thirties, a mother, wife, and professional, I found myself forced to confront the eating disorder for the first time since college. During our walk, I was overcome with unbearable exhaustion. My heart thumped in my chest as I strained to nudge the stroller a little further. At first, I forced a smile to hide this shameful weakness, this failure of a mother I had become. But it wasn't long before even the effort to pretend became too much to maintain. My legs threatened to give out, and my upper body slumped over the top of the stroller. I looked my husband in his eyes, desperate and defeated. *This is not okay. This is not fair to my family. I must banish this demon.*

## A Relapse in the Making

My husband and I were in our midthirties when our first daughter was born. Adjusting to the life changes that come with caring for an infant was challenging, especially for me. Sleep deprivation, overwhelm, and a general sense of disconnection from myself began to settle in. I no longer went to yoga, a practice I had begun during graduate school, rarely did I see friends, and I was too tired to spend time with my husband.

My slowly declining physical, mental, and emotional health during this time in my life set the stage for an eventual eating disorder relapse. I was first diagnosed with anorexia in college, and at that time I received inpatient treatment followed by years of various levels of care and therapy.

After my second daughter was born, the eating disorder came back with a vengeance. After the stress and trauma of pregnancy and giving birth, I now found myself the mother of two little ones, and the anorexic belief system took merciless root once again. As I held my precious daughter in the hospital, I was filled with all the mother's love possible, but a sinister drive to drop the baby weight as fast as possible rang in my head. Old "food rules" returned, dictating what, when, and how I ate. I slowly began to eliminate foods from my diet and cut my intake. This was the only way that I knew to cope with all I was experiencing and feeling. "I'll just flirt with a low-grade eating disorder. Nothing clinical," I told myself.

While on maternity leave, I walked with the girls at least twice a day, an hour each time—the newborn strapped to my chest and her big sister in the stroller. I found the hilliest, most challenging routes possible. "Just a low-grade eating disorder," I'd say, fooling myself.

Breastfeeding kept my restriction in check, as I would never risk jeopardizing my daughter's health and growth. When I stopped nursing at eight months, however, all bets were off. I spiraled into severe restriction, and before long, the last remnants of vitality vanished before my family's eyes. I was so painfully lost to myself. What was initially an effort to take the edge off overwhelm turned into a total collapse of my spirit. The emptier my body became, the more fragmented I felt—torn between unintentionally dying in the name of surviving the weight of overwhelm and my absolute heartfelt desire to be whole for my children and husband. But my time was up. It was do-or-die time. Thank God, I chose *do*.

With the compassionate support of my husband, that Mother's Day I made the hard decision to enter treatment. Initially, I resisted inpatient treatment for fear of abandoning my children and burdening my husband. But partial hospitalization (day treatment) proved insufficient, because I was still dealing with the daily stressors that kept the eating disorder going strong. I needed to completely immerse myself in the healing process, go through refeeding, and (re)learn how to cope in healthy ways.

I was admitted to residential treatment three weeks before my daughter's first birthday. I also committed to completing various levels of care and outpatient treatment for an extended period after the residential program. My intention for treatment was to banish this demon that burdened my family and threatened my life.

Sure, all of this sounded good. I was on the right track, committed to go to treatment to get better. But in truth, I harbored such awful shame and self-loathing. These words that characterized me—anorexia, eating disorder, relapse, recovery, starving, restriction—were all so embarrassing and reinforced my belief there was something in me that had to be banished. Getting "better" was one thing. Believing my existence was anything other than shameful was another.

# My Yoga Story

My yoga journey began in 2001 while I was in graduate school. As an English literature PhD student, my world revolved around words, dissecting language, and communicating clearly—skills that would serve me in unexpected and powerful ways long after my graduate school years.

As I satisfied my passion for learning in my graduate program, another piece of me resurfaced that had been sidelined. An athlete all my life before the eating disorder, I found myself longing to reconnect with physical activity. With exercise addiction in my history, finding a "safe" activity that didn't instigate a drive to overdo it, burn calories, drop weight, and ultimately abuse my body was the real challenge.

With yoga booming in the United States during this time, I decided to join the millions of others and order a few yoga videos. I quickly fell in love with Baron Baptiste's power yoga videos (on VHS!). This more fitness-focused practice was just what I needed to get hooked—to meet me where I was in my search for a renewed connection with my athletic identity. Eventually, I found the courage to attend a class at a yoga studio, also Baptiste style. It wasn't long before this yoga studio became my core community and the asana practice a space for healing my relationship with my body in ways that I had not expected or known I was seeking.

The physical practice coupled with purposeful breathing and core yoga philosophy concepts like non-judgment and compassion guided me to slowly but surely let go of the belief that for activity to count I had to beat up my body or change it. I valued my yoga community and practice so deeply that I began choosing to enjoy these experiences over the narrow world of eating disorder behaviors that depleted me. I craved feeling energetic rather than empty.

By learning how to move purposefully, breathe with intention, get quiet, and purely observe rather than judge, yoga helped me learn how to simply be with my body again and cultivate appreciation for the wisdom of its natural rhythms. Studying ahimsa, or nonviolence (kindness), enlightened me to the harsh realization that eating disorder behaviors and thoughts are violent. I had never made that connection before—that starving my body and overexercising were violent actions. This new awareness motivated me to practice self-kindness. Little by little, I shed the violent behaviors that had once seemed so natural. My yoga practice gifted me with resilience, and I lived in a strong recovery for many years because of it.

## Recovery Interrupted

I completed my yoga teacher training in 2002 and taught for six years before getting married, starting a career, and having children. With life in full swing, there just wasn't enough time in a day to work full time, raise a family, and get to the yoga studio to practice or teach. At the time, I couldn't predict the consequences that would emerge from giving up my connection to the yoga community and this precious time with myself on the mat. The absence of this anchor in my life opened the door for old coping skills and self-defeating beliefs to unsettle the foundation that had held strong for so long. With self-connection no longer a priority, the relapse was inevitable.

Treatment provided the time and space I needed to deeply reflect on what I needed to put in place in my life to maintain wellness. Integrating a yoga practice back into my life was at the top of the list in big, bold letters. In therapy, I identified that dedicated time for self-connection on visceral and energetic levels was crucial for my ability to maintain recovery and nourish the energy it would take for continued healing as I navigated my many life roles. I realized I needed space and time to reignite the creative and intellectual energies that had become dormant as I strove to balance being the "perfect" mother, wife, and professional. Instead of perfection, my mission after treatment was to channel my energy into drawing on the wisdom of my healing journey to help my children have a healthy relationship with food and their bodies. As painful as it was to leave my girls for a month, I am exceedingly grateful to have come home with such a clear and direct vision for how to transform suffering into a calling for the benefit of my daughters.

Time away at treatment also motivated me to change the direction of my career to fulfill a longtime nagging feeling that there was more for me to do in this world. Until treatment, I had never given myself the space to consider what that something else could be. Now was my time to honor the pull of this nagging sensation on my soul. Working with a life coach helped me to create a plan to eventually leave my job as a medical writer. I returned to practicing and teaching yoga and registered for a three-year yoga therapy training program at YogaLife Institute near Philadelphia.

My intention for attending this training was to deepen my knowledge of yoga, satisfy my deep love of learning, and begin a new career as a yoga therapist. Yoga therapy calls on the practices, philosophies, and tools of yoga to support others in making changes in their lives. Unlike a group yoga class, in which all the students follow a sequence led by the teacher, yoga therapy offers an individualized experience. Using yoga therapeutically to empower individuals to create meaningful change in their lives was deeply appealing to me. Plus, this new career was a concrete, unique way to apply my many years of teaching and practicing experience. I knew I was on the right track with yoga therapy, because the nagging feeling—that deep-down hunger for more—had finally disappeared.

## Healing Realized

It was during the three-year yoga therapy training at YogaLife that I discovered my brightest, most whole, and most resilient self. Efforts to "recover" were transformed into a spiritual experience of healing. Comprehensive education in yoga philosophy, yoga psychology, anatomy, biology, and neurology, plus the practices of yoga poses, meditation, breathing, relaxation, and more opened up in me a pure willingness to go into the deepest, darkest, most reticent corners of my being and study myself through the lens of yoga. Learning core yogic philosophies and principles provided me with new language to apply to my recovery and life. From the yoga philosophies of the *koshas* (layers of being) to *kleshas* (hindrances of the mind), *chakras* to *gunas* (both about energy), to the *yamas* (observances) and *niyamas* (restraints), I was inspired with new ways to understand my behaviors, reactions, thoughts, and patterns. The yoga practices of breathing, asana, meditation, visualization, relaxation, and mantra served as the pathways to establishing new patterns and offered me the continuity of self-connection that nourished healing on the deepest of levels.

From this healing work flowed a fuller awareness of my dharma: to support others in eating disorder recovery through yoga therapy. To be honest, this was a calling I hadn't quite seen coming. Who was I to help others in recovery? After all, I was still working on myself. Meditation and conversations with mentors revealed this truth: if there was anything I was going to be an expert in during my lifetime, it was eating disorder recovery. I had over twenty years' experience at this point, and my eyes were fully open to the healing potential of yoga for serving others who struggle with eating disorders as it had me. I set my mind and continued healing to wholly embrace my purpose, and I haven't looked back.

## Embodying Wholeness

A guiding principle of Comprehensive Yoga Therapy is that we are naturally whole individuals. Yoga therapy is a space where we learn we are not broken and that our challenges are opportunities to excavate wisdom. This means we are not our diagnoses or pains or narratives. Rather, we are whole human beings having human experiences.

Learning this concept of innate wholeness was positively life changing. For decades I was preoccupied with my diagnosis and the shameful parts of myself that I identified as broken or not good enough because of the demon called anorexia. How could I be whole if I had something horrible within myself, yet separate from me?

Now I clearly see that the very association between mental illness and "demons" that resides in the social consciousness is one of the greatest barriers to one's healing. I've heard others speak of the devil, evil, monsters, and other forms of possession. I've even heard this language used by medical professionals and reinforced in therapeutic settings. This kind of language keeps us forever unwhole and unwell. It also breeds self-doubt and corrupts hope. How different might my journey have been if I was taught anorexia is a teacher, not a demon? How would your personal journey have been different if you were introduced to this idea?

In the spirit of wholeness, I chose (and challenge my clients) to respect the thing I call my demon as a teacher. Rather than demonize our coping mechanisms, we can learn what they are so desperately trying to teach us. When reframed this way, recovery is a process of searching out the very personal wisdom that the illness holds to uncover beliefs, assumptions, and narratives that require our attention. It's the difference between striving to banish a demon and embracing one's inner wisdom. The former is aggressive and reproduces social representations of mental illness, including that of eternal suffering. The latter is a practice of compassion that empowers one to identify as a human being worthy of possibilities.

My yoga practice and studies guided me to reorient my relationship with my diagnosis—the demon—and to embrace this perspective of wholeness that was so appealing and held so much hope. Central to my process of becoming whole was a critical analysis of the language that I and the eating disorder community commonly use. So much of the shame I carried was related to words like *relapse, slip up, backslide*, and others that connote regression or trigger feelings of failure. According to this lexicon, to *struggle* signaled backward motion, which only fueled a sense of fragmentation and powerlessness to the stronger demon inside of me. To align myself with wholeness, then, meant to redefine struggle as a manifestation of a committed effort to healing. In this sense, struggle is progress, not regression. The wisdom within our struggle speaks to us in the quiet moments of our yoga practices, from which we can be empowered beyond measure to create change in our lives.

Purposely saying "the eating disorder" instead of "my eating disorder" helped me shed the diagnosis identity, reminding me that I am not an eating disorder, or any diagnosis for that matter. Another key change I made in my language is by referring to recovery as a "healing path." I use the words *recovered* and *recovery* mostly because these are so common, but I recognized in myself and in conversations with others how sometimes those words induce insecurity or confusion and even a sense of failure. *Recovery* can feel like such a mountain and *recovered* can feel like a destination. "Healing path" allows me to feel more in process as a whole person.

I've experienced beautiful resilience from consciously revising my language to embody wholeness. Attention to words has become a daily practice, making me more mindful of how language that fragments wholeness versus language that supports it translates into my mood, energy, choices, relationships, and continued healing. My message to clients and others I work with is to find new ways to relate to yourself through language, particularly language of food and body.

I believe we all have a powerful opportunity to shift out of shame into resilience by choosing not to perpetuate self-negativity and other feelings that reinforce fragmentation. With practice and commitment, we can consciously model language that supports our own healing and the wholeness of others.

## Gratitude for the Gifts and Lessons of My Transformation

I've become empowered to transform the wisdom of my experiences to help my children have a healthy relationship with food, their bodies, and self-expression. As a yoga therapist working with others in eating disorder recovery, I have unique insights and tools to offer that allow my clients to reorient themselves to their diagnosis, freeing themselves of the burden of the belief that they harbor a monster inside.

On social and cultural levels, through speaking, writing, and training professionals, I passionately and actively call for a shift in our dialogue about mental illness from one that depicts crippling lack to one that encourages inquiry, self-study, and openness for personal growth and healing.

How grateful I am for that difficult day in the park. I've been fortunate to learn many lessons along my healing path to wholeness. I am no longer ashamed of my past with anorexia. Instead, I am now open to receive the gifts that have come from diving deep into the discomfort and coming out on the other side whole and resilient.

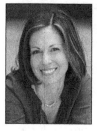

Jennifer Kreatsoulas, PhD is an author, international speaker, and certified yoga therapist. She presents, writes, and leads workshops, trainings, and retreats on eating disorder recovery and body image. She also provides yoga therapy online and in person outside Philadelphia. Visit her at www.yoga4eatingdisorders .com and www.jenniferkreatsoulas.com.

Author photo by Lori Maguire Photography.

# COMING HOME TO ADAPTIVE YOGA

## *Mary Higgs*

As an educator and lifelong seeker, I believe every challenge has the potential to make us stronger, more resilient. If we stay open and curious, each adversity can offer an opportunity to learn, adapt, and grow. But my philosophy was tested when I was nineteen years old. I survived a life-changing car accident, was diagnosed with a spinal cord injury, and was told I would never walk again.

It took years to heal my wounded mind, body, and spirit. The physical and emotional trauma of the wreck numbed my senses and led me to disconnect from my body.

Before the accident, I felt invincible. I was physically strong and never gave up on my goals. I was a dancer, swimmer, lifeguard, cheerleader, choreographer, and athlete. I knew who I was and what I wanted to do with my life after high school: go to New York to become a choreographer and dancer on Broadway.

After the car accident, I awoke to a devastating blow. I had a crushed spinal cord with partial paralysis, and my life was forever changed. I felt alone and lost. My Broadway dreams were shattered. When you're a dancer, your body is your instrument, and if that instrument no longer plays as it once did, your connection to it is broken. It's very easy to feel ungrounded.

## The Rehab Paradigm as Curse and Blessing

When you have a spinal cord injury, numbness or lack of sensation occurs in various parts of the body. In my case, I don't have sensation in several places below my hips, knees, and feet. While this was difficult to accept on its own, the car accident also left me emotionally paralyzed.

I remember the moment my emotional paralysis took root. It was three weeks after the accident; I was on bedrest. Doctors gave little hope for recovery. They tried to prepare me for life in a wheelchair or limited mobility, but I was resistant to everything back then. I not only felt ripped off for my circumstances, I had no idea how to move forward.

Since there were no rejuvenating shots for spinal cord injury patients in the 1980s, Harrington rods were installed in my back to stabilize my spine in preparation for physical therapy. (The rods were removed two years later.) I was also fitted with a body brace that had to be worn 24/7 (even in the bathtub). Needless to say, my day-to-day reality was bleak. Living in my imagination was my savior. I started journaling to calm depression and negative thoughts. It was my life raft.

What little confidence I started to feel a few weeks after the accident was quickly destroyed during a surprise visit from one of my doctors. His cocky demeanor and prickly personality rubbed me the wrong way. He was detached yet overbearing and he walked with a pious, overconfident "I'm above you" saunter.

I felt his uncomfortable gaze as he stood above my bedside and glared down at me for what seemed an eternity. When he finally broke silence, we locked eyes and he asked, "How does it feel to know you'll never walk again?"

His words sent shock waves through my body. My heart pounded. I was furious. I shot him a disgusted look as my face flashed red. He had to have sensed my outrage; I was nineteen and scared, barely able to comprehend what a life of limited mobility would look and feel like.

My fragile state got the best of me, and my words spewed out like a volcano. I leaned forward, shook my finger at his bald head, and let him have it. "You're an asshole. Fuck you. Get out of my room!" I screamed repeatedly until he abruptly turned on his heels and stormed out.

My shrill voice echoed down the hospital corridor, but I didn't care. I felt righteous anger in that moment.

"How dare he?" I cried to my mom, who tried to comfort me afterward. "I haven't even started physical therapy and he was already saying there's no hope and I should give up."

Giving up wasn't in my nineteen-year-old vocabulary. In one short encounter, I felt discriminated against, humiliated, and shamed. I wondered if my doctor did this to every teenage spinal cord patient. The answer didn't matter. My shame morphed into defiance, which I carried into physical therapy and turned into motivation.

When I arrived at the physical rehabilitation hospital, I did everything asked of me and more. I worked on my own before and after physical therapy sessions—sometimes three or four times a day. I was determined. Doctors kept repeating that I needed to accept that I would never walk again. They warned that high expectations would do more harm than good. They tried to get me to socialize with other young car wreck survivors, but I wasn't interested. My only goal was to fight against reality with every physical means possible.

"Your body has been deeply damaged, and your spine will not heal," doctors and nurses said several times a day. "The best way to move forward with your life is to heal your mind and forget about your body."

"Forget about my body?" I thought to myself. I mulled over this sentence and wrote it in my journal. I knew doctors were trying to protect me, but somewhere in my being I knew their advice and concept of healing was wrong.

As a former dancer, I knew the healing power that could be found in the whole-body experience. I understood the joy of feeling my body move. Dancing made me feel alive, and it gave my life purpose. It made me feel strong and capable. Though I have always believed our bodies hold the secret to healing, I wouldn't discover the mind-body connection on a profound level until I found yoga more than thirty years later.

During my time in the rehab hospital, I desperately wanted to prove to myself and my doctors—especially my insensitive neurologist—that

I was stronger than my physical body. I wanted to prove that I could will my recovery. After a four-month stay in a physical rehabilitation hospital, I had more than a year and a half of intensive outpatient physical therapy. By some miracle, I learned to walk again with the help of forearm crutches, a cane, and foot orthotics. Though I had made much progress, my journey came with setbacks and many disappointments.

## Trauma Can Dampen the Human Spirit

Underneath my protective armor, I desperately wanted to blend in. I coped with the emotional and physical pain by hiding my depression. Most days I asked myself, Who am I if I'm not a dancer or an athlete? What was I supposed to learn from this traumatic car wreck? What was God's purpose in putting this challenge in my life? The answers alluded me. I was lost.

Sometimes, strangers would walk across rooms or parking lots to ask, "What happened to you?" Instead of sharing my experience, all I wanted to do was run away. As a result, my anger was so out of control that my boyfriend (now husband) and I derived a solution to deal with nosy strangers. We decided one way to curb curiosity was to slide a hand down to my side and flip the bird to unsuspecting onlookers; therefore, if someone glanced down at my leg braces, they would get a middle finger for gawking.

I realize this was a passive-aggressive, immature response to my own inadequacies. I was young and ill-equipped to handle the road ahead. My negative attitude also demonstrates how feelings of loss can dampen the human spirit. My once bubbly personality turned into self-loathing. I beat myself up for a lack of self-compassion.

My righteous anger lessened over time and it eventually pushed me toward healing. This didn't happen overnight.

Gradually I found the courage to own my body, in both present and past forms. It took years to learn that a strong will or ego doesn't always equal a strong mind and body. It took even more time to uncover a deeper understanding of myself and my health challenges.

Adaptive yoga was one catalyst. It taught me to go within and reconnect mind, body, and spirit. More importantly, I discovered hope within trauma and loss. Pushing my body brought external strength, but I didn't find whole-body healing until I looked within. I now understand a different kind of strong.

## Finding Adaptive Yoga

For a long time, I dreamed of trying yoga, but doctors warned it could reinjure my spine and erase progress. While their advice was meant for my safety, it mostly instilled fear.

When I thought about yoga, I imagined able-bodied skinny girls standing on their heads, bending and stretching in every direction. Going to a studio also felt intimidating because yoga is generally practiced barefoot, and I needed my shoes to walk. I didn't want to feel judged or marginalized for limited mobility. In short, my preconceived ideas about yoga kept me from trying it.

I was fifty-one years old when I finally gained the courage to take my first yoga class and doing so was one of the best decisions of my life. My self-consciousness didn't change immediately, but I eventually found my place. I no longer felt embarrassed about not being able to do handstands or backbends; I no longer worried about not being able to take my shoes off in class. Instead, I sat in a chair and modified or adapted any poses that put a strain on my body. Yoga felt natural in my body. It felt like home, and I felt free.

And once I experienced adaptive yoga and began adapting poses to fit my body, I wanted to share this practice with everyone—especially those with physical challenges. I knew there must be others who could benefit from experiencing this practice. This led me to adaptive yoga and to attend the first Accessible Yoga Conference in Santa Barbara, California.

Attending the Accessible Yoga Conference was life changing. Meeting others on a similar mission—bringing yoga to everyone regardless of ability or background—was inspiring. We were activists bound by our goal to change perceptions of yoga and to make its practices and teachings accessible for all. We wanted to create a yoga community that embraces everyone.

## Adaptive Yoga and Social Justice

In my view, adaptive yoga and social justice are perfectly aligned. Anytime you choose to adapt a yoga pose, you're making a conscious choice to choose movement that feels good in your body. While making choices in poses is empowering, there are many barriers that keep people from trying yoga. I've experienced yoga discrimination at a couple different studios in my yoga journey. After reflection, I slowly peeled back the layers of each instance and attempted to use the humiliation to propel me further in my journey, but making this choice wasn't easy. I share my journey to cultivate change in the yoga community but also to broaden diversity for disabled yogis like myself. I spent years running away from my truth and not wanting to call myself disabled or wanting to be visible in the world. Once I embraced this truth and accepted my body, the world opened up and my authentic voice emerged.

## Finding Yoga, Finding Authenticity

My car accident continues to stretch me beyond my growth edge. I now speak publicly about things I'd kept hidden. While I was once embarrassed to embrace my injury, I now use my life and embody my experience as destiny. Accepting my truth deepened my relationship with my body and improved my self-esteem in new ways. When trauma and loss occur, it may feel like the end, but these instances can open our world and lead to our destiny. They push us into uncomfortable places and provide growth opportunities.

As I step into fullness as a disabled adaptive practitioner and certified yoga teacher, my life has come full circle; I feel like a choreographer and dancer again. In my adaptive chair yoga classes, I build on traditional yoga poses but also use exploration as a way to free practitioners from the rules of yoga. I encourage students to explore their bodies and find what feels good. When students discover they are the experts in their own bodies, they find more self-compassion and acceptance, which are two important goals of yoga.

## Breaking Through My Comfort Zone

Meeting the unexpected is the best part of my life these days. I crave these opportunities. The more I stretch and move past my comfort zone, the more fulfilled I feel. Confronting my fear of visibility and being willing to show up in the world as my full self still feels terrifying. But when we embrace the uncomfortable and connect with the truth of who we are, we can trust what comes up. Our life unfolds if we go within and accept what we find.

While I'm able to manage living with partial paralysis and walking with the aid of plastic braces on both legs, my spinal cord injury and car accident changed and improved my life in unexpected ways. These experiences made me resilient and led me to deeper meaning and purpose. I gain comfort knowing my path will continue to evolve. I thrive in this space. I'm grateful for every step.

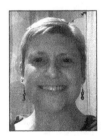

Mary Higgs, MA, is a respected writer, speaker, and empowerment coach. She is an active disability advocate as well as an RYI, OYI, and certified Yoga for All and Accessible Yoga teacher. She loves sharing her message that transformation comes from within and that yoga is for everyone. Mary's work has been featured by Yoga International, Devata Active, Yoga and Body Image Coalition, and Mind Body Solutions. Visit her at YogiAble.com.

# FROM PAIN TO EMPOWERMENT

## *Sarah Garden*

At age eighteen, scared and feeling alone, I sat in a hospital bed waiting for the results of my surgery. I had bruises beginning to blossom on my belly and a welt the size of a baseball just above my pubic bone. During my surgery the doctor sent a nurse to inform my mom that the surgery was going to take longer than anticipated. Finally, when the doctor arrived at my bedside, he informed me I had endometriosis.

After eight and a half years of chronic pain, I finally had some answers. Pain was not unfamiliar to me; in grade two I had been diagnosed with hereditary migraines and by grade five I had chronic pelvic pain that escalated to debilitating pain and vomiting every month when I got my period.

These years were a time when my body and the pain I experienced were totally out of control. I had no agency over my body or my care, and as a result I felt like I had no dignity. As well as having no say in what was happening, I was often told what was happening was all in my mind. I had no control over my body or my pain in addition to having no agency over my treatment and no tools to help me manage. Hormone treatments were never effective, the painkillers I was prescribed rarely helped, and I had no other helpful skills. Beyond this, other than my mom, I was totally alone.

The diagnosis gave me confidence that the pain I had experienced was rooted in this disease. Endometriosis is a sometimes silent, sometimes very loud disease that effects one in ten women, and it can be very hard to get diagnosed. The average time to get a diagnosis when the main symptom is pelvic pain is seven years and four years when the primary symptom is infertility. I was just slightly over the average time frame for diagnosis. Getting a diagnosis is particularly difficult for younger women.[6]

So much has changed since then. In 1990 I discovered yoga and dabbled a little bit. It was one of the only opportunities I had to connect with my body. In 1998 I began to practice more seriously, and shortly after that I had my second laparoscopy. For the first time in over a decade, I started to notice my pain levels decrease. Yoga therapy helped me develop a sense of agency over my body. I was empowered to take charge of my health. I discovered tools that helped keep my body and my breath calm even in the face of pain. I learned how to move again without fear, and my pain started to improve. I also met many other people who had managed or improved their pain and even some people who had eliminated the symptom of pain through yoga. There was even a fellow practitioner and teacher who had used yoga to help manage her severe endometriosis. It inspired me to dig deeper into the practice and start training to teach.

## Shelby's Story: The Role of Empowerment in Health and Healing

I have now been a yoga therapist for two decades, and I see so many people who, like me, lost their sense of agency over their body and health. This last year I got to work with a woman (I will call her Shelby) who has struggled with chronic pain for three years. After fighting her

6. M.S. Arruda, C.A. Petta, M.S. Abrao, and C.L. Benetti-Pinto, "Time Elapsed from Onset of Symptoms to Diagnosis of Endometriosis in a Cohort Study of Brazilian Women," *Human Reproduction* 18, no. 4 (April 2003): 756-759, https://doi.org/10.1093/humrep/deg136.

way through an illness that put her into a coma, she resurfaced with unrelenting pain. Three years of doctors' visits and the main treatment she had been given was opioids, a Band-Aid to mask the symptoms but not a diagnosis and definitely not a long-term treatment. When gathering her history, I discovered she had been to her doctor every couple of months over the course of three years and had never been given a blood test, nor had she been referred to a neurologist to get to the root of the problem.

Shelby had been effectively disempowered by her medical care. I immediately recognized this as the same thing that happened to me.

But once I had a diagnosis, I felt like I had an understanding. I was able to put a name on what I was managing. I was taken seriously, and even though the diagnosis didn't make the pain better, it helped me to better understand and make choices that were appropriate for what was happening in my body.

Yoga empowered me to tune in to my body; it helped me to recognize that my whole body wasn't painful. I am so grateful that I had teachers that encouraged me to choose my practices. Through a decade of feeling like everything was out of my control, choosing what practices felt appropriate for my body and being asked to reflect on those practices enabled me to feel like I had found some personal agency.

In the time it can take to diagnose, treat, and manage illness and pain it can become easy to question your experience, develop a feeling of hopelessness, become isolated, and develop fear around the potential outcomes. This is not to say that these things don't happen after diagnosis, but before diagnosis there is often anxiety around diagnostic potentials and also no clear path to treatment.

After an hour and a half of talking, Shelby and I developed a gentle yoga plan. We discussed potential plans for agency and personal advocacy to get to the bottom of her health. Since then she has returned to her doctor, requested blood work, gotten a referral to a neurologist, and subsequently been diagnosed with a brain tumor.

Now Shelby can move ahead with treatment. She can work to develop a plan to take charge of her health. Even though there is no cure for her tumor, the treatment can help with symptoms and her quality of life can improve significantly. Much like me, Shelby developed pain when she was young. She was unsure of how to advocate for herself and even a small amount of agency created big changes for her.

Taking charge of your own health can take many different forms, but finding health care practitioners that actively listen, believe, engage, and help to co-manage your health can help you build trust with your body and your health care plan. It isn't always necessary to have a health care team, but often multiple practitioners can give you more choices for treatment plans. Sometimes, however, a sense of empowerment can come from building awareness, trusting your body's feedback, and developing tools to help you manage your health.

When I started to practice yoga more seriously in my early twenties, I started to notice small changes. I was so blessed to have found some yoga teachers who used yoga as therapy. Even though there was no direct knowledge of treating endometriosis, they used the approach of meeting each student where they were and adapting the practice to fit the individual and their needs. I started to notice a little less pain with each period, and beyond that I had learned how to change my breathing and the tension in my body when I did have pain. Little by little I learned techniques that allowed me to take charge and feel dignified in my body again.

## Joan: Developing a Tool Kit

In my current therapy practice I work with a lot of breast cancer patients. One of the side effects of lymph node removal is called lymphedema. When you have lymphedema, you develop swelling because the lymphatic system can't process the amount of lymphatic fluid that is being produced. In other words, the system has a certain capacity, and as long as the load doesn't exceed the capacity, there won't be any swelling, but when it does and it is left untreated, it can be devastating.

One of my students (we will call her Joan) was done with her primary breast cancer treatments, and a year later she was excited to make her family Christmas dinner. This was a tradition she hadn't been able to participate in the year before due to her chemotherapy. Joan woke up early to prep the turkey and start to prepare the meal. She had been busy preparing in the days leading up to this and had gotten a little run down, so she was fighting off a cold, but Joan was determined to make dinner this year. Joan spent the day laboring over a hot stove and was surprised to notice that at the end of the day as she sat down to eat that her hand was a bit swollen and her arm felt heavy.

Joan had developed lymphedema. A little over a year earlier Joan had fifteen lymph nodes removed in her breast cancer surgery. This removal made the capacity of her lymphatic system lower. The lymphatic system works to help rid the body of toxins and other waste. It also plays a role in immune function. If the load is low the lymphatic system can process the load but, in this case, she had exceeded her new lower lymphatic capacity. Joan hadn't rested, she was fighting off a virus, she was working hard, and she was in the heat. These are all things that increase our lymphatic load. Joan's newly reduced lymphatic capacity was unable to process the increased load and she developed swelling.

So many times, this can happen to us not just with our lymphatic system but in our body and mind. You can think of things increasing the load on our bodies and minds like stress, trauma, injury, disease, and so much more. At any moment your system has a fixed capacity. As long as the burden of your load doesn't exceed your capacity, you can usually maintain your health. When the load does exceed the capacity is when we usually start to develop health problems, pain, or both.

The good news is that our capacity is changeable. Even when you have lymphedema there are strategies that you can use to make your system manage the load better: manual lymphatic drainage, diaphragmatic breathing, gentle twisting, rest, etc. You get the picture. The same is true for managing illness and pain. We need to build a toolbox that helps us manage increased stress (lymphatic or otherwise), and we also need to develop better tools to help us adapt to the changes in our body or in our environment.

What I didn't realize was happening as I began to dive into a yoga therapy practice was that I was developing a toolbox that helped me manage stress. I was working with my body, breath, and mind to maintain a calm, steady demeanor even in the face of stress. Not only that, but I was learning how to adapt better to changing circumstances. I was slowly and systematically being introduced to movements and practices that I previously never would have thought I was capable of. That was being done in an environment where I felt safe with people I trusted. Without knowing it, I was developing a toolbox to help me increase my capacity to manage the load I was dealing with and an ability to adapt to new obstacles that were in my path.

As I took charge of my health and learned new skills to help me manage my endometriosis, chronic back pain, and the stress that accompanies chronic illness, my community of support started to broaden. We know that social support and love increase survival rates in cancer patients,[7] and research shows that people who are managing pain do significantly better and have lower pain levels.[8] It is not surprising that when we feel supported, we feel safer. When we feel safer our nervous system can stay calmer, and when the nervous system is calm our pain levels can decrease. If the role of pain is to get us out of danger, we are more vulnerable when we are alone.

Just like I developed a tool kit, Joan developed a tool kit that combined yoga therapy as well as regular lymphatic support from her physiotherapy team. We worked on developing a greater awareness of her potential lymphatic load and mindfulness of when her body was telling her to rest. Joan also uses diaphragmatic breathing, gentle twisting, moderate movement, and self-drainage. She has far fewer lymphedema flare-ups because she has a better understanding of what can cause them, and when she does get a flare, she has a tool kit that helps her with treatment.

7. Courtney E. Boen, David A. Barrow, Jeanette T. Bensen, Laura Farnan, Adrian Gerstel, Laura H. Hendrix, and Yang Claire Yang, "Social Relationships, Inflammation, and Cancer Survival," *Cancer Epidemiology, Biomarkers & Prevention* (April 2018): n.p., https://doi.org/10.1158/1055-9965.EPI-17-0836.

8. Jo Cavallo, "2019 Supportive Care: Anxiety, Depression, and Low Social Support Are Significant Factors in Cancer Pain Intensity," The ASCO Post, Harboreside, updated November 1, 2019, https://www.ascopost.com/news/october-2019/anxiety-depression-and-low-social-support-are-significant-factors-in-cancer-pain-intensity/?fbclid=IwAR1KH03fiGtnqxlnI_YTsu8h36UwkGZkr6bOD9wCFQsQRMlK7igg0W1zff0; Eric Jaffe, "Why Love Literally Hurts," Association for Psychological Science, January 30, 2013, https://www.psychologicalscience.org/observer/why-love-literally-hurts.

## Bob: Resiliency Through Support and Community

Support became integral to me as it has for so many of my students. That is one of the reasons I try to encourage yoga therapy students to join group classes. A safe space to share our experiences, a common experience, and support can be so helpful. Early in my career working as a yoga therapist, I had a student who came to class whom I will call Bob. Bob had severe chronic back pain. He had been through four failed back surgeries, and the surgeons refused to offer him a fifth. He came in, talked to me about feeling hopeless, and shared with me that he had considered suicide. Bob lived on his own and had been on disability since his injury eight years before he arrived at my class. Bob's case was complex, and his doctor had not cleared him for much in the way of movement.

After we had chatted for a while, Bob decided he would be willing to try a small group class. In my group yoga therapy classes, everyone does their own therapy practice and I am there to help facilitate. During his intake assessment, Bob told me he no longer slept for any significant period of time and that when he did, the quality of sleep was poor. Our goal was to help him find new strategies to rest and, hopefully through that process, improve his pain. Bob started coming regularly to class. He was slow to warm up to the other students, but they always welcomed him. As he came more often, I began to notice that Bob would get into a supported position and almost immediately fall asleep. He began to use class as his opportunity to sleep.

Bob eventually told me that he felt safe with all the other students and with me. He hadn't thought he would be accepted in a yoga studio because he showed up in his "farmer clothes" and hunting hat. His pain slowly improved, and eventually Bob felt well enough to move away to be closer to his kids. I can't overstate how happy this made me. Bob was not pain free, but with the support of a community, he was well enough to move to have more family support. He told me that he no longer thought about suicide. Support and community can look like a million different things. Sometimes all you need is support.  That may come from one person, it may be a support group, or it may be the love of your family.

I have been navigating endometriosis for over thirty years now. I am happy that I am almost completely pain free. I have to stay active in the management of the disease or I notice an increase in pain again. Through taking charge of my health and developing agency in my treatment and approach to the disease, I can keep the symptoms at bay. In spite of the fact that I have stage 4 endo and I was supposed to be infertile, I was blessed with two beautiful children.

I have an arsenal of tools to manage almost anything that has been thrown at me. Those tools are not only yoga and movement but have also included dietary changes and knowing when Western medicine can be an asset. Through managing my own illness and supporting others in their pain and illness, I have a community of people who support each other and me. I would never say that I am glad that I have endometriosis; a life without it would have been much easier, but I can say that in the face of this disease I have become stronger, more compassionate, and more resilient.

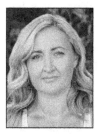

Sarah Garden is the director of Bodhi Tree Yoga Therapy and co-director of Bodhi Tree Yoga College in Regina, Saskatchewan. She runs busy yoga therapy classes primarily aimed at people suffering from pain, womxn's health issues, and cancer. Her classes are fun and educational with an emphasis on healing and re-integrating the body to produce healthier and happier yogis.

Author photo by Shawn Fulton Photography.

# HELLO ANXIETY, MY OLD FRIEND

## *Amanda Huggins*

I remember the first time I experienced anxiety.

I was fourteen, lying awake in bed, tossing and turning as I replayed an interaction I'd had with a grammar school friend that day. While the exact details of the scenario are fuzzy, I remember holding a deep-rooted feeling of being judged (which, for a teenager, is one of the most horrifying feelings in the world). That fear of judgment—and worse, not knowing what to do about it—kept me up all night. I tried to sleep, but every time I closed my eyes, my mind found another opportunity for analysis. Four a.m., five a.m., six a.m. ... my eyelids finally grew heavy, but by the time my brain had become utterly exhausted, I heard a familiar knock on my door. "Sweetie, it's time to get up!"

*What* was *that last night?* I wondered.

Anxiety.

And it would be far from the last time it paid me a visit.

### It's "That Feeling" Again

Sleepless nights like that one didn't become an immediate trend. I wrote about it in my journal and brushed it off as "that feeling." The concept of anxiety wasn't remotely in my vernacular at the time.

"That feeling" would come back now and again during my college years. I quickly learned that other people experienced what I sometimes felt too: unshakeable self-doubt, momentary sadness, and deep feelings of separation from others.

I also learned that in college drinking culture, "that feeling" was often referred to as the "Sunday Scaries." I was told it was normal to feel that way—especially after a long night of partying—and I shouldn't make a big deal out of it. Naturally, I conformed. I bottled up my emotions, continued drinking, and hoped my pesky anxious thoughts would subside. So began the rift between my mind and body.

My behavior was patterned and not atypical from many of my peers: go to class, go to the bar, wake up the next morning, feel anxious. Lather, rinse, repeat. What I once referred to as "that feeling" quickly became a normal part of my everyday life: a familiar (albeit unwelcome) friend.

Subconsciously I always knew something wasn't right. This was more than just a moment of sadness or an occasional ping of fear. What I was feeling seemed deeper, more pervasive, and I struggled with understanding how it could be considered so normal.

*There's got to be something else going on here. Why isn't anyone else talking about this stuff?*

I'd find myself thinking about "that feeling" on occasion but just as quickly tell myself there were much more important things to focus on—like getting a job after graduation, figuring out my living situation, and, of course, finding a cute outfit for that theme party coming up.

The truth was, I wasn't ready to look much deeper.

## You Can Run, but You Can't Hide

Years passed, and I eventually came to learn that "that feeling" was called anxiety.

*Anxiety? But ... I've had a good life. I have no reason to feel like this.*

And there it was: my first of many attempts to brush off the depth of my feelings. *I have no reason to feel like this* was code for *I'm afraid to take up too much space. I'm afraid to express myself.*

In the earliest stages of understanding my anxiety, I found myself falling into deep guilt when I'd attempt to claim my experience. I've always been aware of my privilege—I'm a white cisgender female, grew up in a stable household, and have been blessed with loving friends and family—so acknowledging anxiety as a major part of my story felt shameful.

*I have no right to feel like this,* I'd think. *I just need some sort of change.*

In an effort to escape my anxiety, I packed up my bags and moved to San Francisco where my worst nightmare was realized: not only had my anxiety followed me, it had become exponentially worse. My journal entries at the time, which started out filled with awe and excitement for my new city, quickly devolved into shame-riddled ramblings about my emotional discontent.

*Well … it's a Friday night and I'm staying in because I'm feeling completely horrendous.*

*My anxiety's coming back again, and it's actually pretty bad. Worse than ever, maybe. Last weekend it literally kept me up at night. I can't tell anyone about it either because I know the act of explaining it will just give me more anxiety.*

Nothing had changed. There I was, a twenty-something living in San Francisco who still couldn't shake "that feeling" from when I was fourteen. That's when I realized that while I wasn't ready to talk about my anxiety just yet, I needed to try *something* different.

Enter: yoga.

## Meeting My Triggers on the Mat

What was most jarring during that time was that, despite so many years of being deeply unhappy, I still had nothing to show for it. No answers. No lessons. I *still* couldn't figure out why I was so anxious.

So I decided to put my analytical mind to work and began a survey of my life. While there were countless potential and existing triggers, I found three main themes:

- *I was certifiably in a financial crisis.* I had maxed out all of my cards, was living in one of the most expensive cities in the US, and was working fifty hours a week at a job that barely allowed me to pay my rent, let alone pay down my debt. I would then try to numb the stress by going to the bar, which only drove me deeper into the hole.

- *I wasn't entirely comfortable in my skin.* I was at odds with my body, moving between different disordered eating patterns in another attempt to numb out. I remembered reading an article that spoke about "being in your body," and I had absolutely no clue what that meant.

- *I wasn't quite sure who I was.* Beyond the physical connection to my body, my soul was aching. The person I tried to show the world was completely different than the person I *felt* I was. Rather than seeking clarity, I had spent months on end battling with myself.

The list grew longer, my self-awareness began to deepen, but I still couldn't crack the code. I was certainly learning more about myself but was emotionally still numb.

So I shook things up by checking out a yoga class down the street. It wasn't my first yoga class, but it *was* the first class I'd ever gone to without friends, and I was SCARED.

Why? Because going to a yoga class—by *myself*, no less—brought up absolutely every anxiety trigger I'd ever experienced:

Money: *I have to pay how much to rent a mat? And a towel?! This better be worth it.*

Independence: *I'm by myself. Do I look like a friendless loser?*

Judgment: *Oh my god. Is that person looking at me? Do they think I suck?*

Perfection: *I can't look like I don't know what I'm doing!*

Body Image: *I'm not as thin as the other girls here.*

Had I realized all of that at the time, I probably wouldn't have gotten out of my bed that day to go to class. But *something*—an intuitive hit, perhaps—guided me there that day.

I wish I could say that from that class on I fell in love with yoga and we lived happily ever after. Wouldn't that be sweet?

But I HATED that class. I was infuriated that we had to hold poses, bored during *savasana*, and I just didn't "get" the whole breathing thing. Above all, I couldn't believe I had allowed myself to spend a full seventy-five minutes staring directly in the eyes of everything that triggered me. Yoga was horrible! Confusing! Hard! I vowed then and there that I would *never* go back.

Until the next day, when I went back to that very same class, just to make *sure* I hated it.

And the next day too ... just to be *extra* sure it sucked as much as I thought it did.

And then, of course, the day after that, I tried out a new yoga studio ... just to compare the sucky-ness of it all.

*I'm just doing my research,* I thought, in an attempt to downplay the fact that my developing yoga practice was becoming a playground for exploring my anxiety.

## How Movement Helped Me Heal

A few weeks later, I was beginning to fall deeply in love with my yoga practice. My anxiety, my triggers, and my fears were as present as ever, but for the first time in my life, it felt safe to begin exploring them.

Yoga gave me what I had been searching for all along: the reconnection of my mind, body, and soul.

In the months prior, I had been working diligently on exploring my anxiety using only my reptile mind: I would make lists, I would analyze, I would think ... but I had never allowed myself to get into the depths of my emotions.

It finally clicked during a particularly powerful practice one rainy afternoon. I had started going to a donation-based bhakti studio in San Francisco, where classes began and ended with collective song (something that would have terrified me only months prior). For perhaps the first time ever, I caught myself *singing*—not whispering, not mouthing along to the words—but *singing*. Completely connected to the words, to my practice, to myself. I was allowing myself to feel without judgment.

In that moment, it hit me: it wasn't enough for me to simply *see* my anxiety, I had to feel it too. I had to connect my analytical mind with my heart in order to heal.

On my mat, I discovered a place where I could explore the darkest corners of my mind without fear. All of the things I was afraid of looking at—my imperfections, my flaws, my sadness—were fair game, and I was ready to play.

I think my favorite part about the process was how completely different each practice was. Some days, I was reeling in this never-before-felt confidence, this vibrant sense of joy, this newfound ability to feel.

*Oh my god, I can feel. I can FEEL!*

Other days, feeling was overwhelming, and I'd find myself crumpled in a puddle of tears.

*Oh my god, I can feel ... everything.*

It was the juxtaposition of my own emotions in which I started to unearth the deeper beauty of the practice. Yoga is a process of constant change. A practice of fluidity. In that understanding, I started to realize that there wasn't much of a difference between my "good" and "bad" days; what mattered most was how I chose to show up.

I kept coming back to my mat. I became a patient observer of my thoughts. And what I loved the most was how my reactions to my triggers were beginning to shift:

Money: *I'm becoming more comfortable investing in myself.*

Independence: *Going to yoga alone is actually pretty rad.*

Judgment: *Even if someone is looking at me funny, do I really care anymore?*

Perfection: *I kind of like when I mess up. At least I'm learning.*

Body Image: *I didn't know my body could do this!*

In that process of re-patterning my thoughts, I began to recognize on a much deeper level that the root of my anxiety had to do with a denial of who I am at my core. I am an expressive, feeling, passionate, and imperfect being, and I had tucked away those critical parts of myself in an effort to avoid judgment. There had been so many different points in my earlier years when I had been told I was "too much." Too sensitive, too emotional, too weird, too loud—the list goes on. As an adolescent completely unequipped to stand up to those judgments, I acquiesced ... but I never lost those parts of myself. They were simply hidden away, fighting their best to be heard and seen, and using anxiety as the vehicle to let them out.

Through my practice, I began to understand that the judgment I had felt was unavoidable because it came from within. My anxiety wasn't about being judged by others; it was born from the judgment I held for myself.

Anxiety is the thoughts, feelings, and sensations that result from your inner world and external world living in conflict.

I recognized this key truth on my mat, and I resolved to find meaningful harmony through befriending and accepting myself.

## From Practice to Purpose

After almost two years in the Bay Area, I headed south for Los Angeles to follow an unexplainable call to relocate. I didn't consider myself fully "healed" yet, and I wasn't *quite* sure what I was looking for when I left, but I knew I'd figure it out once I got there. I leapt and the universe was there to catch my fall. Within a few short months of settling into my new home, I began a yoga teacher training program that transformed my life. The deeper I dove into my practice, the deeper I dove into myself.

The unfolding of my self-study was beautiful, but it wasn't without road bumps. In addition to deepening my yoga practice, Los Angeles brought a new way of life, new friendships, and new relationships— many of which reactivated some of the deepest triggers that I hadn't yet created the space to feel into.

Now that I was finally *allowing* myself to feel, when those deepest triggers became realized, I felt them hard. There were months when I felt even more disconnected from myself than I did when I was in San Francisco, but now I knew what to do about it. I had tools, mentors, and my practice to hold space for me as I worked through some of the most difficult parts of my story. While the work wasn't always easy, it was always worth it.

I look back on my struggles with anxiety and now see them as the greatest blessings of my life. The pain, confusion, and judgment that I experienced were all necessary for my growth and finding my purpose.

Through deep inner work (and the guidance of my mentor and dear friend Melanie Klein), I ultimately left the corporate world to follow my call to become a coach. I didn't know of any other anxiety coaches at

the time to model my business after, but I *did* know that I wanted to become a resource for those who felt just as lost as I once did. With that as
my north star, I have become deeply committed to those I serve, helping them step into the most empowered versions of themselves.

I think fourteen-year-old Amanda would be proud.

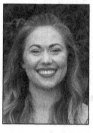

Amanda Huggins is an Anxiety Coach and founder of
Anxiety to Empowerment LLC. In addition to private
coaching, she creates anxiety management programs
and online videos that are distributed worldwide. She
has appeared on numerous podcasts and online shows
and at in-person events to bring her method of healing and personal development to those who need it
most. While Amanda works with clients around the
world, she currently resides in New York City.

Author photo by Jhana Parits.

# WILL I EVER TEACH YOGA AGAIN?

## *Sarah Harry*

In 2017 I fell on a concrete floor, broke my kneecap, and discovered I had irreversible, incurable osteoarthritis (in many parts of my body). That entire year I worked and worked on my yoga and physiotherapy practice to strengthen, heal, and chase the pain away. But one morning I put my feet on the floor to get out of bed and I sobbed in agony. Yoga just couldn't heal me.

I am an Australian yoga teacher in a curvy body, a psychotherapist, author, and activist, and I work for myself, so any threat to my livelihood is a worry. Even though I knew I always had my career as a therapist to support me, I love teaching yoga retreats and workshops to help people heal their relationships with their bodies and disordered eating. I didn't become a yoga teacher until later in life—forty years old—so there was still so much more I wanted to give.

Yoga is a practice of eight "limbs" or parts, and those include breathwork, meditation, and single-pointed concentration to name a few. *Asana* is the word we use for the physical practice. I suppose I most often spent my practice on asana, meditation, and breathwork, but I didn't want to lose any of it.

So I followed the medical path and a surgery was offered to me: a risky, painful surgery with a 50/50 chance of success.

There was a question in the air for me. Much more important to me than the odds of the surgery, but I didn't ask my surgeon the question when we met. Or pre-op, or post-op. I asked at the final check-in. I was still in pain, but the surgery was successful. I held my breath.

"Will I ever teach or practice yoga again?" I finally exhaled and let the words hang.

And his casual response no way matched the gravity of the question. "Oh, well, no. Not really. You will never kneel or bear weight on that knee again and probably best not to. I wouldn't risk it."

Then he stood up, all smiles, and said he hoped he wouldn't see me too soon (I will need another surgery but hopefully not for many years), and before I could blink, I was paying, leaving, and in my car. His words settled on me like dust and heartbreak.

For the next month I grieved, and I meditated, and I practiced *pranayamas* (yogic breathing techniques), so yoga didn't leave me. But I longed for the fluid moving and stretching component of my practice. To have back what I had taken for granted. Effortless practice. Not perfect. But perfect for me.

What I didn't know in the grieving weeks was that it wasn't over. There was more to come. A month after the surgery, after the "all clear," it got worse. So much worse. One ordinary Tuesday, I lost the use of my legs. It was a slow-motion collapse, an almost graceful sinking to the floor.

I was in my kitchen when it happened. Somewhere inside of me fired "danger," and my arms went out to catch a nearby bench so that I wouldn't land on my damaged knee.

For a moment or two I held the bench. And I am a fat yogi, so this was no mean feat with my legs no longer working and the pain beyond comprehension. Inside I heard the words "get to the ground." So I did. I lowered myself onto my stomach, feeling a mix of agony and a strange sense of my legs not really being there.

I was strangely calm. I don't know in what order, but I figured I would get some post-knee-surgery painkillers and pick up my kids from school. It took an hour for me to drag myself on my stomach to the phone to call a relative and ask for the medicine, but I realized I was in denial. I was immobile. Almost afraid to breathe. I called an ambulance instead.

They sent two very burly ambulance drivers, "ambos" we call them. I don't think they were ready for my total immobility. The one in charge got down on the floor with me. "Mate, you are going to have to stand up; we have a slide thing at the stairs, and you're just going to have to make it to the stairs." That would require me to take six steps maybe.

I remember just looking at him. I never say, "No, I can't." I'm pretty agreeable. I'm the strong one. The one you want in a crisis. With the first aid certificate.

"I can't," I said, looking him square in the eye.

"Plan B then," he said. He must have seen that look before.

Plan B was something called "the green whistle." I had no idea what it was, but they said, "Breathe in," and I inhaled from the "green whistle," the opiate they gave me to get downstairs, and I quickly lost consciousness.

I don't remember how I got downstairs, but from the look on my mum's face when I asked her later, I don't think it was elegant.

I came to on my street on the gurney. I still couldn't move, but I was really happy. Then, according to my neighbor, I asked for my phone so I could take a selfie with the ambulance driver. She refused, completely horrified. This was fortuitous: later, my drug cocktail would lead me to post a whole lotta stuff online that I could have kept to myself.

I was admitted to the hospital quickly and rolled slowly into the MRI machine to diagnose my lifeless legs. I had ruptured four disks in my back pretty badly. Turns out they don't send you home to look after your kids if you can't walk. (I am a single parent.) Thank goodness for my mother, who supported me then and always.

About seven hours after falling, I was in an uncomfortable bed in the oncology ward. Not ideal, but there were no beds anywhere else, and at that point I was so happy to be safe and relatively pain free. I have a traumatic relationship with pain. I know that some time in my childhood or young adulthood something happened. I don't know what because, like sometimes happens with trauma, I have sealed it off really tight.

However, it was enough for me to refuse a natural childbirth in 2006 out of sheer terror and anxiety for no reason I or anyone else could make sense of. I had nightmares about the pain, vivid and terrifying, escalating the more pregnant I became. So finally my gynecologist, happy enough to have a predictable birth to schedule, gave me a date to bring my child into the world. Pain free. It was the most calm, joyful, and wonderful experience.

But then several weeks after giving birth I had two experiences of extreme pain, just weeks apart, which added trauma to trauma and caused me to carry a deep fear of the way my body can both make a baby and whip around and render me breathless in agony.

I drove myself to the hospital with acute appendicitis and a fresh caesarean wound (excruciating and dangerous). My appendix burst as they wheeled me into surgery. And at the time I didn't even know what I was having surgery for. They were moving so fast they had forgotten to tell me. Later the surgeon told me it was one of the worst cases of appendicitis he had ever seen. How had I driven? My ability to withstand pain is mixed with my fear of it.

Three weeks after my appendix burst, the same thing happened to my gallbladder. Post-op, I was in a small suburban hospital when something ruptured. No physician was willing to come see me on a Friday night, and no one was authorized to give appropriate pain relief. All I remember was the nurses saying, "Stop screaming, you are upsetting everyone."

I wasn't a screamer before, and I haven't been one since. So it must have been bad. In the morning I was vindicated by the surgeon, who was horrified to learn what I had lived through. It kind of didn't matter then, though. The nurses' shifts had changed, and the slow drip of pain medication finally eased into me.

That was twelve years ago. I had yoga then, but it was only a basic physical practice. I was strong and young; I don't remember really learning about the other beautiful parts of yoga. Just that I could do a handstand. I was a student, not a teacher. Still, I found it a haven, a healing space. It didn't take me long to hit the mat after my surgery. I went to class whenever I could get a willing babysitter. But still, I didn't know there was this huge amount of yoga I was missing. I just wanted to get my strength back!

At the time of my fall in 2018, I was a yoga teacher with hundreds of hours of training. I had all the tools I needed to use my practice from the moment I opened my eyes. I just had to remember and stop feeling sorry for myself. After my collapse, I stayed in the hospital until I was stable, then went to inpatient rehabilitation, then day-patient rehab. All in all, I spent nearly a quarter of 2018 in a medical facility. At first, I was on so many drugs that not a single element of yoga crossed my mind. When I got to the rehabilitation hospital, I asked my mum to bring in my mat. It looked at me for a long time, unused in the corner of the room. I knew I couldn't walk; they wheeled me in on a gurney. Someone showered me. I was very, very sad. But the rhythm of the rehabilitation the specialists put together was soothing, predictable. I allowed myself to look at the mat in the corner every day and one day, some sparks finally fired.

At first I really didn't want to practice yoga at all. I was too raw, angry, and depressed. But there was still a lot of time to kill, and my mat, sitting there in that corner may as well have been a neon sign: Yoga has eight limbs! You still have so many ways you can practice!

It was bed yoga first, practicing some of the movements lying. It was too hard to do any meditation or breathing with my mind foggy from medication. I did anything I could manage lying down with the help of my team.

My first question to the physio who designed my rehab program was, "Can I do yoga in the water?"

"I will make you a deal," she smiled. "If you do the program and you have time when you finish, I will teach you some safe yoga practices to do in the water."

HA! Did I have time? Yes, I had time. You have never seen anyone move as fast as I did. My legs moved through the cleanest, warmest, most luxurious water. In the hydro pool I was weightless, but I knew. I knew I would be able to walk on land again. Even though on land my treatment team was confused. Was it my knee? My back? I kept collapsing, even with support. I called it "giving way."

Which leads me to *savasana* (lying relaxation), meditation, and pranayama. The trilogy that I began practicing almost every day. Even the movements I did privately in my room began to change. Slow, in bed or a chair, upper body mostly, then moving my legs.

I arrived at rehab on a gurney, and six months later I walked out. But most days I questioned if that was going to be the case. Clichés were the hallmark of my stay: "You can do it," "Don't give up," "Just a little bit more," "We will have you up and like new in no time!" The staff cheer-leading, demanding, faultless, and kind.

Really it's just grit, pain, and exhaustive repetition. But I had yoga and toward the end of my stay, gingerly using the very sturdy armchair to lower myself to the floor, I could finally use my mat again. I used every pranayama I had ever been taught; I meditated through exhaustion and pain. I got better faster than they thought because of my practice.

I am careful, and I am terrified of falling every day still. No one really knew how hard it was and how many times I wanted to give up and stay in the wheelchair, then on the crutches, and then finally with the limp. But with luck and the support of an incredible medical team, I did it.

I still do rehab every day, including hydrotherapy. I have pain in my knee and my back most days. I will never walk up or down stairs with ease. Mostly I am on my mat with my bolsters and cushions and special knee ball. But I show up for something. Anything. I think I have become more graceful as I've slowed my movements down.

And my knee surgeon's prediction?

I went back to teaching a few weeks after returning home from the hospital. I wasn't being cavalier or reckless. I just listened to my body and frankly could see no problems in starting slow. So I did.

First I taught sitting in a chair, then I moved to two crutches and fi-nally one, but I will never teach like I used to. I don't demonstrate every pose. I have a chair with me at all times. None of my students mind the changes; they see me as the same slightly irreverent, inclusive teacher I have always been.

There are many ways to share yoga with others. So what if I will never do another salute to the sun or rest on my knees! My heart ex-pands with the fact I can show my students—when they feel tired or they're injured or lacking an ability in a certain area—what they can do with the magic of a chair, wall, prop, or just the ability to know themselves well enough to reach into the eight different limbs of yoga and find one to nourish them.

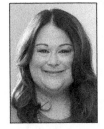

Sarah Harry is an Australian body image and eating disorder specialist, registered group and individual therapist, lecturer, and yoga teacher. Her passion is making yoga accessible and breaking the mold of the "yoga body." She is the author of the book *Fat Yoga* and the founder and director of Body Positive Australia and Fat Yoga Australia. Learn more at www .bodypositiveaustralia.com.au.

Author photo by Lucia Ondrusova Photography.

# PART TWO: REFLECTION QUESTIONS

- When you consider showing up as your full self and allowing yourself to be visible, what emotions and sensations arise for you?
- How has the practice of yoga supported you in remembering your capacity to thrive?
- How has your practice created a space for you to practice more self-love and compassion?
- How would you like to begin honoring your innate wholeness?

—Michelle C. Johnson

# PART THREE

## *Moving Through Grief and Loss*

How do we overcome the universal yet so very personal pain of loss: loss of loved ones and loss of aspects of our identity? This question is unpacked in various ways throughout this section, where the writers share how they've navigated the rough terrain of grief, along with the resolutions they found along the way. Although every loss cannot be reconciled—some are too shocking and unimaginable to ever accept—we can find a balm of wisdom within to carry us through even the most tumultuous directions in life.

That wisdom often comes through presence, but presence is hard to find in trauma's wake. Learning how to be "here" after loss was a conundrum Kathryn Ashworth faced after years of struggling to process the violent death of a close friend. She coped by fighting with her pain in various ways instead of softening into acceptance. Ultimately, it was through an introduction to yoga and the healing wave of her own breath that she began to thrive—instead of only strive—and regain a sense of wholeness in the present.

For Tonia Crosby, loss came in stages: first her father, then her support system, and eventually, her health. After the death of her father and subsequent decline of her family, she lived with chronic stress from an early age and later battled with breast cancer. Through her practice, she found both the external and internal support she needed to not only survive cancer, but to also transform long-standing pain and awaken a sense of magic and playfulness in her life.

Sarah Nannen experienced the unspeakable pain of losing her husband while raising four young children. With this loss came the expectations she set for herself to be the "right" kind of widow and mother and to be the person who overcame the odds. She developed the habit of running from her pain, quite literally, in marathon after marathon. But through discovering a mindful practice more suited for her, she embraced stillness and a life on her own terms after loss.

Loss also lives in our bodies. As a survivor of sexual trauma, Zabie Yamasaki carried a painful experience in her body long before she delivered her firstborn son who was stillborn. It was through raising her second child, a healer in her life, that she stepped into a practice that served as a salve for the loss. Her experience as a mother, combined with yoga, helped her recover from her traumas, uncover a resilient and caring relationship with her body, and develop a yoga therapy network of support for other survivors.

Networks of support are vital, especially for underserved communities. Through her recall of growing up in a Black community in South LA, Alli Simon reminds us that healing is a collective effort and often a matter of privilege. After travelling the world, she became even more aware of the racial and geographic divides that create barriers to wellness, but through yoga found a "backdoor" to healing. Through a devoted practice she was able to heal from the loss of her sister, father, stepfather, and best friend (among others) and then committed herself to making this resource available to everyone.

And of course, the incremental practice of letting go is essential for stages of grief to unfold. Using the science of epigenetics and wisdom of ayurveda (a system of traditional Indian medicine), licensed professional counselor Kathryn Templeton shares how grief, trauma, and joy are passed down intergenerationally. Through a case study and telling of her own family history, including the loss of her father, she shares how making the unconscious conscious can help us create new imprints that lead to healing and a greater understanding of where we've been.

# MEDITATION

## *I Am Fully Alive*

For this practice, if it is comfortable, please move onto your back. If being on your back would feel uncomfortable, then please find a comfortable posture and set yourself up so you feel supported with props, pillows, blankets, or whatever is available to you right now.

We will start with a breathing practice to quiet your mind.

Close your eyes or soften your gaze and breathe into your body. Start by taking deep breaths in and out. You might even place a hand on your belly and a hand on your heart and breathe for a few minutes, noticing the rise and fall of your chest as you inhale and exhale.

If it feels safe, bring your awareness to the experience of grief and loss. You might think of someone or something you have recently lost. You might think about a relationship that has changed form or shape. You might think about the loss of a beloved or fur baby. You might not think of one particular event but instead the experience of grief and loss in your life. If it doesn't feel safe for you, you can think about your experience of witnessing someone who has lost someone or something.

Breathe deeply. Breathe into the space where grief lives; breathe into your heart space. Notice emotions as they rise and fall. Notice memories as they move through your mind and spirit. Allow yourself to feel the full range of emotions related to your experience of grief and loss.

Stay here for as long as feels good to you.

When you feel ready to move out of meditation, take a moment to thank your heart and breath for supporting you. Take a moment to honor your experience of being fully alive, which means being with joy and suffering. Take a moment to attend to any tenderness that is present, knowing it is okay to be tender. It is okay to feel.

Bring your awareness back to the hand on your belly and the hand on your heart. Bring your awareness to the room you are in by gently opening your eyes wider and reorienting to the space, noticing colors and any sounds in the room. Take your time, and when you feel ready, roll to one side. Take as much time here as you need before gently pressing up to a seated posture. As you feel ready, move out of your seated posture and gently move about your day.

—Michelle C. Johnson

# LEARNING TO BE HERE AFTER LOSS

## *Kathryn Ashworth*

I've never felt like the most mindful or centered person, and I certainly never intended to become a yoga teacher. And yet I am one. It's a strange thing to admit perhaps, as generally such a decision is made and carried through with thoughtful planning. But it would be this inevitable stumble into a career—rather, life path—that led to my greatest healing.

The story of how I got here begins at an unassuming yoga studio tucked away due to lack of noticeable marketing or word of mouth—a small studio that reflected warmth, clarity, and humility in its design. Nothing flashy about it. Nothing outwardly indicated that so much was about to change for me. I wouldn't have even noticed it existed had I not been seeking a job and saw a front desk position advertised in my local paper.

The plan was to attend a yoga class after I dropped off my resume, which I knew would be different from the yoga I'd known. I'd been practicing hot yoga mainly for about a year and before that spent time at an ashram (spiritual community), which I'd visited as a new, idealistic college graduate.

Most importantly, this was also a time of grief, when I was struggling to admit that one of the most beautiful people I'd ever known had been shot and killed—gone in an instant. It still hurts that I never got to say final things to him, including how much he meant to me. But we were teenagers when we knew one another, experiencing a phase of life that felt sweetly infinite. Moments were savored but also taken for granted; there was time but there *really* wasn't.

He was eighteen when he died, and I was seventeen. Now, at thirty-two, I've lived nearly twice as long as him.

Looking back, I realize now that when I entered that studio space, I was seeking more than a job; I wanted to keep my feet in yoga circles however I could. I felt the answer to my pain was there, in yoga—and at twenty-five, after years of holding on to my grief, I needed one.

After talking with the staff and subsequently learning that they weren't hiring, I walked into the practice room to lay out my mat. But instead of seeing single file rows of yogis that I could neatly fit my-self into, everyone was sitting in a circle wearing street clothes with notebooks in hand. This *wasn't* going to be a yoga class. Before long, I realized that what I'd really walked into, was, well, a teacher training informational session. Though I could have sworn the schedule I'd read online said otherwise—that it was a "free" community class.

So there I was, a newish yogi in a room full of aspiring teachers. It was awkward but also oddly intriguing. I wasn't super familiar with some of the most common yoga poses yet, including downward-facing dog (the Bikram sequence, a standard twenty-six poses, doesn't include that one). I had been busy trying to "lock" my knees in forward folds, thinking that was the best way to release tight hamstrings while doing my best to not faint in a 105-degree practice room.

Basically, I had no illusions and knew that I wasn't prepared for this training program, and I suppose the most logical thing would have been to leave that room. Who takes yoga teacher training on a whim? At a studio they only just arrived at? Isn't that dishonest?

But I didn't leave.

And it would be through this training that I'd learn what yoga truly is, at least to me, and gain the tools I needed to release my grief. Let me preface all of this, however, by briefly explaining that when I entered that studio, I still had a very warped idea of what it meant to do both.

## The First Stage of Grief

I can't describe what it feels like when someone you love disappears overnight, let alone due to violence, so for the most part I won't really try. One moment you're able to reach for their arm, and the next, you're running your hands through the air desperately trying to find them. It left me mute. In a freeze state; like an antelope playing dead in the jaw of a lion. And if I could have made sense of what happened in words during the thick of grief, perhaps I could have forged ahead more effortlessly.

When I found yoga, I was deep in the throes of post-traumatic stress, which, from my experience, feels like a world apart from others' worlds; I couldn't reach out to anyone for help, let alone a therapist. So I tried to do it all, all by myself. Pushing myself and simultaneously avoiding myself was the only coping mechanism I could grasp, and I took that mentality into everything I did, including yoga.

At the ashram, I could pretend for a moment like none of what I felt mattered. It was easy because it was a motto this particular *sangha* (community) went by: thoughts and emotions are only distractions. Then, once I began practicing hot yoga, I used the practice to reaffirm that I had overcome those distractions. If I could only reach that ballet barre behind me, as I dipped back into a standing backbend, surely I would further confirm my mastery over them.

It was good that this action made my back hurt and that the goal was impossible. It was an opportunity to not feel what I felt, to bypass it completely as I moved endlessly toward the barre.

When I took a seat in that circle, at that new studio that I knew basically nothing about, all I can say is that something simply compelled me to fold to gravity. The teacher began asking for our names and eventually got to me, and I admitted that I didn't know what I was doing there. But she was welcoming and encouraging, and soon into our brief conversation she asked a question that cemented the deal:

"Are you spiritual?"

"I have been my entire life," I responded, somewhat surprised, as it felt so personal.

"Then," she replied, "you can take this teacher training program."

If spirituality was a foundational requirement for this training program, then perhaps I *could* do it. I've done a lot of praying in my life. I was the only kid in Sunday school class who wore an absurdly large wooden cross around their neck. I also took *too* feverish notes as my teacher talked about Noah and the flood. And during services, when my preacher would say, "If you haven't had communion before, don't just walk up here, run"—well, I ran.

Yes, I'd had communion before.

As a teenager my spiritual inclinations switched from Bibles to tarot decks. The spirit I spoke to was no longer "God," but I still communicated with something higher than myself. A curiosity about another world has been a part of me all along.

So I signed up.

I bought the books and a few more yoga pants. I got a fresh spiral-bound notebook. I didn't look back and I didn't know what I was in for; yes, I'd drawn from the proverbial tarot deck and pulled The Fool card.

The course was broken down into weekend segments for a nine-month period, so I had time to integrate what I learned, which I was glad for. During that time, I also attended regular classes. I was expecting we'd move through some vigorous asana and then learn about postures, but instead the yoga was far more gentle—calming, nurturing even. And to my surprise, it involved a lot of sitting and lying down and breathing.

The day my teacher taught us how to set up a meditation seat, got out her mala beads, and started reciting the *maha mrityunjaya mantra* exceptionally fast is particularly memorable. The maha mrityunjaya mantra I now know is the "death conquering mantra." Although no one really conquers death, it is said to help the practitioner conquer their fear of it. To me, it sounded like a spell, which from my new age, unconventional perspective was pretty cool. It was an indicator of "magic"—something magical to me at least.

I was training somewhere that cared about the rich philosophical underpinning of yoga. As it turns out, the entire sequence we were learning to teach (really, that I was learning to practice if I am honest) was to move us inward toward a "true" self. In psychological terms, one could call that a big self—a whole self, an integrated self. Something I think I'd gotten glimpses of before, in my happiest moments. Like when I was a child, playing in my backyard with my dog. Like every time I've ever seen a sunset. Something that's harder to feel when you're experiencing the fragmentation inherent to trauma.

According to the teachers I'd found on this path, this was something I could learn to get back in touch with on a regular basis—a feeling I could expand and make more pronounced in my life over time, gradually, through systematic practice. And the strangest thing about the practices we explored was that the most profound experiences I ever had were during moments of the least amount of effort.

## Rest and Breathe

One of my current yoga teachers, whom I met years after teacher training but is of the same style of gentle yoga, often says, "If you don't know what to do, rest and breathe." As someone who didn't know what to do for a long time other than strive, this has been a game changer for me.

You'd think that as human beings, we would give our breath some thought—if nothing else, we might feel grateful for it. But I never thought about breath before yoga or even really felt myself breathing; I just breathed. And because breathing is a part of the autonomic nervous system, the beauty of it is that I didn't have to ask myself to do it—none of us do. But it's also an aspect of that system (unlike our organs) that we can consciously shape and control, or perhaps the better word is "guide."

The vagus nerve innervates the torso, and when this nerve is activated, it has a soothing effect on the body and mind. We stimulate that nerve through belly breathing. Try lying on your back; let your body be still (completely still) so that the only part of you that moves is your belly. Breathe through your nose, unless congested, and let your belly rise on the inhale and fall on the exhale. Again your body is still, and most importantly, your chest is still. Over time, allow your breath to become naturally smoother and deeper, and breathe in a way that feels just right for you.

And that's all it takes. It's a straightforward practice that can lead to a pervasive sense of peace. Lying back and breathing is all that's required of you.

This was the exercise we explored in teacher training, among a few others related to breath awareness and training. Our assignment was then to go home and take it "off the mat," to breathe that deep belly breath wherever we went.

I must have been chest breathing the entire way home, because at some point I had to make a conscious shift. This happened in my kitchen while I was washing dishes, and to this day it remains one of the most healing experiences of my life. It was simple: I was there, present, watching the bubbles pop and slide across surfaces—hearing the slosh, gurgles, and clanging of the plates and silverware submersed in water.

## Simplicity Is Not So Simple

"And that's all it takes" was what I'd always wanted to hear. And in moments, there's a lot of truth to a statement such as this. I'd been on hyper alert for years; this moment of peace felt like a lifetime—and that moment gradually built, each peaceful moment connecting to one another. But ultimately nothing is a quick fix.

When you have trauma, it's not exactly easy to "sit with things" because a threat lives in your body. I see now that I was a warrior in those early days of practice, and I don't regret fighting for myself. I also see that I had to believe that I was a skillful one—capable of entering and leaving the battlefield as a conqueror. In that regard, bypass had its time and place for me—so did the ashram and that first yoga teacher whom I met there.

I've been in the slower-yoga game for seven years now and if I am honest, I still find it challenging to not skip the awareness parts of the practice, which I truly have come to believe are the most essential parts of practice.

But I am learning to be here.

## Teaching

It took me a total of three years to complete that teacher training program, which was the maximum length of time anyone could take it for. There came a point in time when I even wondered if I could finish it;

I think that lingering feeling of "imposter syndrome" remained with me longer than I realized.

And truth be told, sometimes I still feel like a yoga imposter—like I just walked back into that room, feeling apologetic for my very presence. But something keeps me in yoga spaces. Something brings me to my mat; sometimes something (an emotion or thought) scares me away from it again. But it's less of a battle now and more of a dance of healing. A dance of compassion and a dance of regret for the times I was less compassionate. A dance of self-forgiveness. Stages of grief unfolding. Now that I have this resource, which I have learned to trust and rely on more and more over time, I am more able to hold space for and process these layers of myself.

Something willed me to start teaching, too.

I now teach a regular class every Wednesday at 5:15. On any given night, four to ten people arrive, and the same core (four) group of women always arrive. At the end of class, I leave fifteen minutes for guided relaxation in *savasana* (a pose that requires no effort and simply involves lying on your back), which is a lot in our busy world. When I first taught it, I wondered if anyone would come back—as they say (and as I've experienced) savasana (read: resting, non-efforting) can be one of the most challenging practices in yoga because it's hard to release control. I also know that because of this, it's deeply gratifying. I hope that they can feel that too and that it provides a thread they can use to improve their days and heal in the various ways we humans need healing.

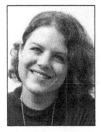

Kathryn Ashworth is a writer, editor, photographer, and yoga teacher with a background in anthropology. She views yoga as a healing resource that can awaken a sense of wonder and individual purpose, and her specific interests lie in simple and adaptable practices that anyone can benefit from. She is currently a senior editor at Yoga International.

Author photo by Patricia Perano Photography

# IMPACT

*Tonia Crosby*

My father died when I was nine years old.

He passed on before my grandparents, or great aunts and uncles, or any of the other elders in my family. It was my first experience with the loss of a loved one, although grief was not unfamiliar to me. My childhood was often filled with sadness and rage. I suppose that is how I understand grief, as the amalgamation of sadness and rage.

He was killed on Easter morning, in a car accident on a stretch of highway we had driven a thousand times. At a nondescript place on the side of the road, between the city and my hometown, my warm, charismatic, protective father's heart exploded in his chest from the impact. He was a cocaine addict. And a heart abused by decades of narcotics use—from Vietnam to my third-grade year—couldn't withstand the head-on collision.

My mother made me go to the annual Easter egg hunt that morning anyway. I will never forget the disbelief I experienced as I watched a man mow his lawn, a woman adjusting the bows in her daughter's hair, and hundreds of smiling children racing around me to gather eggs in the green grass. The memory is so vivid in my mind that even now, some thirty-three years later, I still dream of it and wake weeping for that little girl—standing frozen amongst an entire community, basket hanging limp in her hand and tears streaming down her face, wondering how all of these people could go on like nothing terrible had happened. And no one noticed.

In many ways, my mother went away then too. He was the love of her life, and she would never remarry. But she did spend a decade filling the void. Booze. Drugs. Men. Work. Therapy. She kept a roof over our heads, even if the lights went out sometimes. And she kept food in the cupboards, even if that meant cans of lima beans and cheap hotdogs for weeks on end. But she did not choose us—her children; she was largely unavailable, and we learned to look out for ourselves. I often look back on the years after my father died, and what fills the picture in my mind most is the deep sense of loneliness that permeated our home.

In the absence of healing, a profound and constant sense of lack kept our family from thriving in the aftermath of my father's death. My mother was not equipped to support herself through the loss, much less provide tools and resources for my sisters and me. It became a life lived in continuous survival mode. And so, when other adversity occurred, from my mother's DUI in the next-door neighbor's driveway to unimaginable sexual assault, we simply endured. And the trauma compounded and stacked, layer upon layer, in our internal and external lives, until the best we could hope for was tenacity.

## Endurance

As a teenager and young adult, my choices and behavior reflected a girl deeply hurt, generally lost, lacking much-needed support, and seeking attention. But somehow, I was able to convince everyone around me that I was fine. I have chosen to believe that. Otherwise, I would have to believe that of all the people who claimed to love me, no one loved me enough to see that I needed help.

During a stint of intense therapy later on in life, I was able to pinpoint the place in time when I developed my fiercely independent worldview—a deeply engrained lens that created my unmatched willpower but also the painful belief that no one would show up for me because I was unavoidably alone.

I was eleven years old.

The year after my father died, my mom bought us a boxer puppy for Easter. Surely, she was masking the pain, but I think she also believed we needed protection during her constant absences from our home. And Lady Alison Lavon the Boxer (Ali for short), the unruliest dog on the planet, was protective, to say the least. And so she was home with me the night it happened.

My mother was away most nights, and I was almost always home alone. Still, I was glad to have my dog—she provided a sense of security and unconditional love that I had lost when my father collided with that tractor-trailer.

I was asleep in bed when the rattle of the chain-link fence outside of my window woke me. Immediately, Ali was barking and snarling at the back door. We lived in a seventies-style ranch home with a long hallway leading to the kitchen, and when I rounded the corner to see what was happening, I locked eyes with two strange men standing at the sliding-glass door. As soon as I retreated back around the wall to hide, I realized I had to get to the phone, which was only inches from where they stood. It was the middle of the night, I was by myself, and no one would help me unless I got to that phone.

I still talked to my dad a lot during those years, conversations that kept him alive in my mind. In that terrifying moment, I begged him for courage, and I ran for the avocado-green phone on the wall. Somehow, I made it to the phone and back to the hallway without ever looking at the door, and with the coil of cord stretched as far as it would go, I dialed 911. And the police came. They hunted down my mom at a bar in town, and soon I was sitting at the kitchen table, frightened and exhausted, surrounded by adults that I did not trust. For all the things that were said, and all the questions that were asked, there is only one statement that I remember.

My half-lit mother said to me, "You better get used to it kid. We're on our own."

## Loss

Post-traumatic growth is paradoxical. In the yoga and mindfulness field, we like to assume that resiliency means we have overcome our trauma and thrived as a result. But sometimes, resiliency and the success it breeds come from the survival mechanism—an "I'll show the world that I can make it despite the horrors" kind of attitude. And while this can seem impressive from the outside, it is, more often than not, dangerously repressive on the inside. The repression of emotional trauma happens when we do not have the tools and support we need to heal. And for some of us, this means pushing the pain down so deep, and striving so hard to prove it wrong, that we create disease.

I was diagnosed with stage III breast cancer when I was only thirty-three years old.

There are many folks, in and out of the Western medical complex, who will disagree with what I am writing here. But as an academic-minded woman, who has experienced, studied, and survived cancer—and all that surrounds it—for almost a decade, I am not at all convinced that cancer is simply a disease of the physical body, even as it manifests there. For me, and for countless others with whom I have spoken, cancer is far beyond our meat suit; it is a constant mental, emotional, and spiritual experience of loss:

Loss of autonomy. Loss of hair. Loss of income. Loss of control. Loss of comfort. Loss of body parts. Loss of loved ones. Loss of ability. Loss of appetite. Loss of intimacy. Loss of bank account. Loss of hope. Loss of agency. Loss of vitality. Loss of self-image. Loss of life.

Loss. Loss. Loss.

My first cancer diagnosis occurred while I was a nontraditional adult student in graduate school, studying peace and justice at the University of San Diego. I was on the road to a high-powered career in human rights when a pesky lump in my breast catapulted me home to Colorado for treatment and into a bed in my sister's basement. At the time, I felt like I was losing everything that I had worked so hard for, not to mention the loss of my agency in the face of standardized health care (or what I like to call the cancer conveyor belt), and the likely loss of my hair and breasts and any positive body image I might have had.

I railed hard against the system in the months following my diagnosis. I went toe to toe with doctors and nurses and technicians. I pushed back against the cancer machine that felt draconian and dehumanizing in every cell, healthy and otherwise, in my body. I read countless research articles and dug through every alternative therapy website and book I could find. I devoured patient forums and spent innumerable hours in cancer chat rooms. I was driving myself mad with the will to survive and the confusion about who or what would save me, all the while projecting myself onto the public screen of social media as strong and happy.

It was exhausting to be a survivor. But one of the things I found in all the work of trying not to die was meditation. I had long since practiced what I thought was yoga but was actually gym-style asana calisthenics for a nice ass. And while I heard teachers talk about meditation in those classes, I only recognized its power once I read an article in a consciousness studies publication that described decades of peer-reviewed research about the power of meditation for healing. Of particular interest to me was the role of meditation in the regulation of stress hormones—which have been tied to cancer, hypertension, and all kinds of other diseases.[9]

One of the things that all my tests showed was that my stress hormones were through the roof. And even though a highly recognized oncologist swore to me that my cortisol levels and my cancer were not related, I had a deep knowledge that all I had suffered had come to roost, and that no matter the treatments I endured, I would not survive if I did not do the work of healing from the roots of my pain.

---

9. Rainer H. Straub and Maurizio Cutolo, "Psychoneuroimmunology—Developments in Stress Research," *Wiener Medizinische Wochenschrift* 168 (2018): 76-84, https://doi.org/10.1007/s10354-017-0574-2; Murray Esler, "Mental Stress and Human Cardiovascular Disease," *Neuroscience & Biobehavioral Reviews* 74, part B (March 2017): 269-276, https://doi.org/10.1016/j.neubiorev.2016.10.011.

# Returning

I attribute much of my ability to thrive through the painful experiences of cancer to a mischievous and otherworldly Tibetan physician. In a mystical turn of events, he became my lead doctor—and life's teacher— shortly after my second of five diagnoses. Within minutes of our first meeting, he traced my illness back to the grief, loss, and trauma I suffered following the death of my father and throughout my pubescent years. He made it quite clear that cancer is not the disease but the symptom of the disease—in this case, my complex trauma. And perhaps most importantly, he told me that the journey I was embarking on would be long and difficult but that he would be by my side every step of the way, even if I did not believe it yet.

I will forever perceive that moment as the (re)turning point in my life.

The Doc, as I lovingly call him, prescribes hand-rolled herbs to aid in healing my physical body. But this is only a small part of his care. It is the prescription of yogic practices, spiritual searching, radical self-love and acceptance, and letting go of samskara that have undoubtedly saved my life. The Doc has, over our eight years together, guided me down the path to transformation. But the work, in the form of practice, has always been mine to do.

There have been so many experiences that could have been the end of me since I met the Doc. When my mother died, and my cancer recurred, and I lost my business. When I lost my breast, and chemo wasn't working, and I grieved most deeply for the loss of romance and intimacy in my life. When I lost every bit of comfort and lay awake night after night in excruciating pain, terrified by the drugs and wishing that my life would end. Being told that it would.

Still, I am as alive as I have ever been. And the creation and sustenance of life force in me is a direct result of my practice. For me, practice is the unification of my internal landscape through lifestyle. And that lifestyle is a mash-up—part yoga, part Buddhism, part flawed human.

I use lifestyle to inspire the playful little girl in me—the one who is happiest in nature, who, despite the hardship, always craves exploration, who is incredibly courageous but whose empathy can make her very vulnerable. She practices in the woods on long hikes with her dog. She practices through laughter and silliness. She practices by allowing others to hold her and comfort her. And she loves headstands.

I employ the things I have learned through hardship to ignite the healthy woman in me—the one who knows to go to the mat instead of the bar, values herself regardless of whether a man wants to have sex with her, and nurtures herself with what she believes and deserves no matter what. She practices yin in long, sweaty spells next to the fireplace in the winter months. She practices radical presence during sex. And she shows her love for herself and others through nourishment: crafting delicious meals, baking decadent Bundt cakes, and investing in joyful experiences of all kinds.

And somewhere along the line, I learned to rely on the wise old lady in me: to listen to my intuition, to believe in magic, and to discover and transform the pain—all with the help of a universe much greater than myself. My practices are simple and sustaining because I have learned that this life need not be a fight. I sit, I chant, I pray, and I believe.

I am well into my forties now, and I go on living.

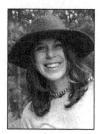

Tonia Crosby is the founder of bhavanaKIDS, an organization delivering award-winning yoga and mindfulness curriculum to young people. She is also a creator and contributor in a number of other projects aimed at teaching tools and strategies for living a meaningful life. She is a cancer thriver, partner, podcaster, animal lover, and a woman who loves to be in the wild. You can learn more about Tonia at toniacrosby.com.

# THE ONLY WAY IS THROUGH

## *Sarah Nannen*

I wanted to be anywhere else.

In someone else's body.

In someone else's story.

*Anywhere* less painful than the wreckage of my own life.

Six days after my beloved husband was pronounced dead at the site of a military aviation accident, I boarded a transpacific flight from Tokyo with my four children, their four car seats, and our eleven bags headed for our new, not-so-temporary stateside residence in my parents' home.

Despite the loving welcome and blessing of so much support, we were moving into a scraped together, surreal reality I'd never choose.

In an exhausted, freshly postpartum, heartbroken body, my days now began with the painful ritual of waking to the nightmare of grief. The first moments of consciousness each morning brought a wave of peace blanketing my awareness. Behind it though, the forced remembering would slam into its rightful place as the details of our new existence played across my mind's eye like a horror movie on the drive-in screen.

*He really was dead.*

*They did actually come to our door on a sunny Sunday to tell us the devastating news.*

*I was truly terrified of who I would become without him.*

In my darkest hour, on top of my heartbreak, came the sense of physical betrayal from my own body. Everything in my body hurt. I was carrying the forty pounds of pregnancy weight left behind in my postpartum body. I didn't recognize myself in the mirror. In fact, I hated what I saw. My breasts were tender, leaky, and operating around the clock, on demand. My heart rate would skyrocket from the systemic inflammation of stress and the pain of my feet on the floor first thing in the morning. My hormones were in a state of chaos that pinned me down with chronic fatigue, my thyroid struggling to keep up, my reproductive system painfully taxed, and my heart palpating randomly, sometimes even at rest. My joints ached. My skin ached. Some days, even my teeth ached.

I finally understood the lived terror of hopelessness.

Yet, somehow, I was feeding the children, keeping the plates spinning, and making huge decisions about our future. Many days felt like an out-of-body experience—watching a stronger version of myself go through the motions of the day from somewhere far away. I didn't recognize my life and I certainly didn't recognize myself in it.

Just months after giving birth and weeks after my husband's death, I did the one thing I knew how to do when life felt out of control: take the control back. Thus began my marathon training plan. Instead of creating the most gentle, quiet healing space possible to nurture my little family into this new reality with the deep healing we needed, I ran for my life.

My nervous system was hanging on by a thread. My body was operating in a constant state of stress. While the pregnancy weight was melting away as I trained, so was any thread of well-being I had left. I wanted to run to escape the overwhelm of my daily reality. Instead, I was running to depletion what was left of my battery.

I kept telling myself that the training was the one thing keeping me stable; I was truly expecting my mental health to be competely destroyed by grief at any moment. The more intensely I pushed, the better it worked, I figured. After all, I knew the experts recommend exercise for mental health.

I pushed my body harder and ran miles upon miles each week, convinced finishing the race would make me feel strong. I cried during so many of those long runs. Not from grief but from fear. I devoted myself to completing a marathon I didn't have the strength to finish because I believed if I quit—if I let the marathon defeat me—everyone would know I had been destroyed by my grief and my *new* worst fear would be realized. I couldn't handle the shame and hopelessness of that possibility.

So, I pressed on, determined to cross the finish line.

I ran that marathon hoping to convince everyone else I'd be ok. But secretly, I was hoping to convince myself I was going to make it. Somehow completing a marathon felt like proof I'd be able to outrun and outlast the unyielding grief. Being seen as "a widow *who can still run marathons*" gave me a stronger identity to hide my pain within. I hoped it might make me immune to the onslaught of well-meaning pity I encountered everywhere I turned.

I thought I'd feel powerful, courageous, and untouchable after finishing the 26.2 miles in honor of my late husband, Reid, with our friends and family cheering me on every step of the way. Instead, I felt frustrated, hopeless, and full of pain the day I finished that race. Surrounded by friends and family who traveled far and wide to be there to support me, I felt more alone than I ever had. As everyone celebrated my strength at the post-race party, my inner and outer worlds collided, and an excruciating truth slammed into view: I was attempting to outrun my pain. It wasn't working.

*Now what?*

I had a marathon under my belt and another one in the works. We had moved out of my parents' place and into our own. I was finding my stride in daily life—the way a solo mother of four finds her stride, that is—counting down the hours 'til bedtime about two hours into the day and operating on sheer willpower, fueled by the constant fear that everything would come crashing down around me if I slowed down even for a moment.

The whole world was constantly sending me the message that I had done it—conquered even the impossibility of grief.

"You're so strong," they'd tell me.

"You inspire me," they'd say.

"I don't know how you do it," they told me over and over.

They meant it as the highest compliment, but their words cut like a knife.

Perhaps on the outside I looked strong. The strength and grace I exuded for public consumption was in direct conflict with the dark agony that thrashed around uncontrollably in my inner world. Every time someone commended me for my strength, I felt strangled by shame and at the same time, disconnected and invisible.

I longed for someone to know my inner truth alongside the strength they saw. I wanted true connection—for my pain to be acknowledged and my fears to be embraced, something I didn't yet know how to do for myself.

Just about a year into widowhood, I started to panic. I was desperately looking for something else to cling to, a last-ditch attempt to scrape together some kind of life for myself in the wake of my beloved's death—to dodge the stigma of widowhood and the devastation and darkness of grief. My postpartum body had regained its strength thanks to the marathons, but the sheer exhaustion was constant and the physiological anxiety persevered. Life felt like treading water in quicksand now. A futile attempt at survival.

That is, until I began a 200-hour yoga teacher training course with Pranakriya School of Yoga Healing Arts based on the teachings of Swami Kripalu and Yoganand Michael Carroll. Beginning that certification, I thought I was filling in the blanks of an empty-feeling life with merely *something to do*. It felt like the next welcome and worthy distraction from the painful truth of my reality. I figured I'd learn the intricacies of yoga postures (asana), a few breathing techniques, and enough Sanskrit to teach a well-polished yoga class or two each week while my kids were at school.

Instead, yoga ignited the flames of healing within me I hadn't been able to access another way. I had unknowingly committed to a powerful practice of vulnerability and presence that would require me to walk into the depths of my grief with tender curiosity so I could begin to heal.

I had begun a journey home to myself that would change the course of my life.

Until that turning point in my life, I had placed the highest value on dodging, weaving, and out-hustling my pain. I had been unknowingly devoted to compartmentalizing—staying just busy enough to be too tired to feel and projecting strength onto the stage of my life. Yet, my teacher Yoganand taught that self-observation without judgment is the highest form of spiritual practice. This deepening journey with yoga invited me to begin knowing my own pain for the first time, and in doing so, begin to know myself.

Walking into the flames of grief opened a way through to something *beyond surviving.*

"Breathe deep into your belly and feel your body expand," he'd say.

*Run,* my mind would respond.

"Be with whatever thoughts come as you hold the posture," she'd say.

*It's too much,* my heart would scream.

"Watch the stories your mind creates about the nonexistent future with curiosity," she'd offer.

*It's not safe to do that,* my thoughts would heave in protest.

And then, I'd stay anyway. I was learning to cultivate my capacity for gentle self-witness. I'd feel my feet on the floor and feel my breath in my lungs and when I did, despite the warnings of my mind to escape this new awareness of what I felt there, I'd find a pocket of peace within myself to soften into. It took me months to even notice what was happening and longer to fully receive it. Even so, learning to access a safe haven within myself allowed me to sustainably continue the practice of learning about myself through yoga and pranayama so that I could continue to heal. That curiosity and ease also carried into my daily life off the yoga mat too.

Some mornings, I'd wake early to attempt one of the personal yoga practices required to complete the program. Instead of forcing my body to move, sometimes I'd light a candle, breathe for a few minutes, and

then lie supine on my yoga mat. I'd release the urge to perfectly perform the flowing movements of asana and I'd allow my yoga to be mo-
tionless. Once a fierce warrior who willingly pushed far beyond my own
capacity and well-being, I had become a woman who was no longer
willing to force myself to do anything that felt so far outside the truth
of my needs just because I was "supposed" to. I rejected the concept of
*should* without apology.

It was terrifying to begin with, yet the willingness and ever-increasing
capacity to be in stillness with myself, my feelings, and my fears is truly
what allowed me to begin my lived experience of healing.

With each practice, I was learning to be with the reality of my
thoughts and needs, some days in total surrender to quiet, others flowing powerfully through asana while connecting my movement to my
breath. I was learning to live fully present, to be with whatever came my
way, to move with life instead of running from it.

I had become a spiritual warrior with true compassion for myself,
not the fabrication of grace I had been trying to force since the day I
learned of my husband's death. The sadness was still there, but the way
I experienced it had begun to shift. It felt less like a catastrophic monster attempting to swallow me whole and more like a love-filled note of
gratitude for the gift of having shared life with him for those fourteen
years.

The full embodiment necessary for these yoga practices asked me to
inhabit my own body and therefore my life from a new state of mindful presence. That meant being with the ache of longing and the overwhelm of life exactly as it was. It meant acknowledging the exhaustion
of my body and honoring the loneliness of my heart. It meant understanding my self-judgment and the shackles of guilt, shame, and fear I
had been imprisoned by in life. It meant holding gentle witness for the
energy I had spent in devotion to being a "good" widow. It meant being
as curious about my fear of forgetting him as I was about my fear of
moving forward.

Yoga was my invitation to experience life after loss more fully alive.
Yoga became a committed practice of self-witness that allowed me to

focus each day on the integration of my inner truths with my outer lived experiences into a more honest and empowered harmony.

Because of this, something really important (and unexpected) happened: I was finally able to think more clearly, and my body began to heal. I became more empowered and more hopeful about my future. I noticed what felt like a bizarre shift in reality—right there along with my grief and sadness existed a deep joy and gratitude within me too.

While it seems like a miracle, the shift I experienced as a result of practicing mindfulness is backed by science. When we experience any painful transition or loss, our physiology moves into an activated trauma state. In a state of fight, flight, freeze, or fawn, our organs and systems begin operating differently because our body's primary objective when stressed is survival. As a result, the sympathetic nervous system is activated and stays on high alert until the threat has passed. This changes the way we think, behave, and react to the world around us.

It doesn't actually matter how technically life-threatening the source of stress is either. If we perceive our existence, reality, or identity is threatened by the stress catalyst, our body responds as though our life is in danger in return. No amount of fake-it-til-you-make-it can overcome that. With grief and trauma, we can't just wait for time to heal all, as the adage goes. Instead, we must choose to cultivate a state of ease in the body that allows the internal state of emergency to be lifted so our physiology can transition back to homeostasis. This isn't a mind over matter switch you can flip. This survival mechanism is deeply seated in our primal brain. Most of us will need professional support and a community standing in solidarity in the trenches of healing by our side to do so. Only when we've helped our physical body move beyond surviving will we have access to the mental and emotional healing we seek.

Looking back, the intense running was keeping me stuck in panic mode physically, which made it impossible to get to work on the painful thoughts and feelings in my head and my heart. It wasn't until I introduced mindfulness practices of breathing (*pranayama*) and yoga (*asana*) that I started to curate an ability to reframe my thoughts away from panic. Not only was I practicing self-observation without judgment, I was also helping my body reset to a parasympathetic state of "rest and digest." And that paved the way for a journey through grief toward a sweetness on the other side I could never have imagined that day in Japan when my life changed forever. My healing began within my body—through yoga and breath. What I found there changed everything. In cultivating the physical capacity to experience the deep healing of ease and presence at a biological level, I had created the conditions required to be safe. That embodied sense of safety inspired my ability to access the emotional vulnerability, intuition, and understanding of myself that was necessary for the mental and spiritual healing so deeply needed in grief to begin.

*Here's what I know for sure: Grief can make you feel invisible. To others, at first, and eventually to even yourself if you abandon what's true for you. There is no healing in disconnect; this is the place of forever pain so many believe is inherent to grief. Here's what I know for sure: grief is an intense journey we move through and the revelations, even more than the loss, will change our lives in powerful ways.*[10]

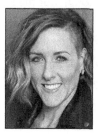

Sarah Nannen is a trauma-informed life coach and transformation teacher, speaker, author, and the host of *The Other Side of Rock Bottom* podcast. Sarah became a military widow and solo mom in 2014 when an aviation accident claimed her husband's life. Her journey through grief informs her renegade work with those navigating painful life transitions who seek to live extraordinary lives. Sarah lives in central Illinois with her fiancé, Brad, and their four children. Learn more at www.sarahnannen.com.

Author photo by Chris Eckert.

10. Nannen, Sarah, *Grief Unveiled: A Widow's Guide to Navigating Your Journey in Life After Loss* (NY: Morgan James Publishing, 2018), 117.

# FINDING SAFETY AMIDST THE STORM: TRAUMA HEALING, MOTHERHOOD, AND YOGA

*Zabie Yamasaki*

The capacity of the human spirit to heal in the midst of the unfathomable is something that continues to take my breath away.[11]

This body has survived sexual violence. It's grown two little boys over the span of a year and a half: one angel who stayed for twenty-six of the sweetest weeks I'll ever know and one rainbow who came into the world in the most peaceful of ways in October 2016. He rewired the immensity of trauma I had been carrying within my body the moment he was laid on my chest...thriving, breathing, and beautiful. Mothering has unveiled parts of myself I never knew existed. We find our way together. He healed the trauma wounds that I held inside, just by his little body breathing on mine.

---

11. This essay was inspired by a piece that first appeared on For Women Who Roar. Zabie Yamasaki, "A Soft Place to Fall," For Women Who Roar, April 23, 2019, https://www.forwomenwhoroar.com/nonfiction/2019/4/23/a-soft-place-to-fall.

My body has also known the most remarkable love—it has felt held, lifted, and supported. Yet at the same time, *I've* struggled to love this body through the ongoing somatic impacts of trauma. But this body is healing, even when that healing is not linear. This body holds light and dark. The past decade has been a series of highs and lows that have undoubtedly shaped the struggle that is resilience, growth, and healing. This journey has been one of deep work to uncover the layers of trauma within every cell of my body in order to find my way to the light. A journey where I am hardwired for connection with many resilient souls and survivors who have helped me navigate the darkness and showed me that I have never been, and will never be, alone. It's taught me to have the courage to embrace the most vulnerable moments of pain, to let myself feel it all, and to never lose sight of who I am and everything I've dreamed of for this life. I've learned that I can grieve but I can also thrive.

## Living Through Loss:
## The Visceral Experience of Grief

I will never forget the moment on June 26, 2016, when the nurse looked at me with tears in her eyes as she reached for my hand and said, "I am so sorry, sweetheart. His heart is no longer beating." I was twenty-six weeks pregnant.

I felt the pieces of my heart shatter inside of me. My heart felt far too small to carry a pain so large. I fell into my husband's arms. The tears turned to numbness. I felt worthless. Our baby boy had died. And I would have to deliver him. The journey to motherhood had wrecked me. This loss was compounded by the way in which I moved through the world as a survivor of sexual trauma: consistently feeling a loss of control, carrying feelings of shame and blame, and feeling like my body had betrayed me.

In the months that followed the passing of my first son, I cried enough tears to fill an entire ocean. I stretched, made art, rested hard, did nothing, sat in silence, felt the sun and let it thaw my grief, let the ocean heal me, read, journaled through pain, went for long walks, held my doggies, asked for help, took many things off my plate, learned who really loved me, let go of guilt, let go of my constant need to over achieve, let myself be taken care of, held my husband tighter, witnessed true heartbreak in my parents' eyes, embraced my pain and vulnerability, and more than anything, I discovered the intensity of a mother's love.

I've learned so much from my complex relationship with grief. Grief is palpable and it is heavy. When you let it in instead of suppressing it, it can teach you things about yourself that you never knew. My grief has revealed the depth of my heart. This pain has shown me that I can put my pieces back together differently. This continues to be a challenging yet liberating practice.

My grief has softened me. It's helped me learn the preciousness and beauty of life. My grief travels with me on my yoga mat and makes its way into each intention I set. It tests me and shows me my strength in the most intense moments of despair. My grief is with me when I smile and when I have innocent moments of joy and peace. Grief taught me that it could exist in my body simultaneously with joy. It reminds me of what I've lost and my capacity to work through. My grief has taught me that healing has no timeline. My grief has taught me that it can coexist with love. And that both are essential to surviving. It's taught me that both grief and love can exist deeply in my heart. And that both are essential to surviving.

There's no getting over. There's getting stronger. On one particularly difficult day when I didn't feel like I could go on, I took a pregnancy test. The two little lines stared back at me, and with pee still on the stick, I ran to the living room to share the news with my husband. Both of us filled with joy and excitement as well as anxiety and fear.

## When There Is Rain, Look for Rainbows

I will never quite know how I survived my subsequent pregnancy after stillbirth. Some days it was like learning how to breathe minute to minute. What I do know is that as I moved through the unfathomable anxiety, I trusted, believed, hoped, loved, and surrounded myself with those who truly made me feel seen.

The moment my second son came into the world was the first day I had taken a real breath in a very long time. My husband placed a lavender cloth on my forehead and three pushes later, with "Over the Rainbow" playing in the background, Hudson made his entrance into this world. Every day still, I just stare at him and think, Is he really mine?

He is my dream come true and my healer. As I reflect now on my very early postpartum days, I remember vividly the cherished nights that turned into days and the days that turned into nights with him falling asleep only on my chest. I would rock him, stare at him, and tears would roll down my face and fall on him because some moments I just couldn't believe he was actually here. I would spend entire days in my bathrobe—face-planting on the couch at 9 p.m. exhausted, sleep deprived, and hungry—only to wake up five minutes later to gaze at photos of him on my phone while he slept. His little smile has expanded the edges of my heart and brought the joy back into my life.

I experienced something I can only describe as magic when feeding Hudson from my own body. Breastfeeding has been a tremendously healing and restoring experience for me. My past traumas have challenged my worthiness, my sense of control, and have made it difficult for me to see my body as a safe and sacred place. There are days I don't really know what "coming home to my body" means when it has been a vessel of betrayal.

The memories are visceral, but he helps me move through the numbness, the lack of connection, and the feelings of blame. He affirms the magic and awe of feeding and nourishing him from this body—the one that has experienced unfathomable pain but is strong and capable of developing new frameworks that are grounded in healing, growth, and resilience. He has helped me reshape this journey. He allows me to realize what my body can do even when it feels weak. And most importantly, he has given the pieces of me that have been pierced new memories.

## The Body Remembers: Reclaiming Healing Through Trauma-Informed Yoga

As a survivor of sexual violence, the years of disconnect I felt from my own body were more than I could have imagined. I wasn't prepared for the way my past experiences of trauma would sneak up on me and manifest in various areas of my skin where painful memories still existed.

Sometimes, triggers would brew and create sensations in my limbs, leaving me with a heavy heart and frustration as I sat in anxiousness at the thought of having to explain these somatic feelings in talk therapy.

I carry my most painful and traumatic experiences in my body. The body remembers. There are still some places that are so fragile and tender that they require extra nourishment, support, and intentionality. Each day is a recommitment to loving myself more fully and paying attention to what my body is communicating to me about what I need. Living with trauma can make it really difficult to access parts of ourselves that may feel frozen, numb, or even too painful to explore.

I spent years searching for a panacea. I suffered quite viscerally from the impact of my trauma. It manifested in overwhelming anxiety, GI issues, flashbacks, nightmares, toxic relationships, overworking—the list goes on. It wasn't until arriving at the practice of yoga that I realized that reclaiming choice with my body was going to be an ongoing process for the rest of my life.

I quickly learned that what I needed was something tangible. I needed access to something that allowed me to feel like I could use my body to regain power and control. Yoga entered my life at a time when nothing else made sense.

It was within the four corners of my mat that I began to realize I could protect my energy and my peace, and I gradually began to embrace pockets of relief in joy—no matter how fleeting. My practice helped me find words for my feelings and also gave me permission to move forward when words could not do justice. The practice allowed me to feel lighter, more balanced, and grounded. It allowed me to take control of my healing in profound ways.

I finally had an outlet to process the unsafe feelings that were residing inside of me. Yoga gave me a form of self-expression that allowed me to move beyond trying to find the words to articulate what I was feeling. Yoga has helped me stand in my light and find my voice despite all the ways trauma makes it easy to feel small. Yoga reminds me each and every day that I am more than the darkness that was done to me.

It has played an instrumental role in the journey of finding a safe home within myself.

My practice has showed me what it means to be a steady and safe anchor amidst the many storms that surround my life. I used to brace myself for the next wave to crash. Now I've learned to rely on those inner tools to help me be brave. It's shown me my strength when I convinced myself I had none.

Yoga can certainly never take away anything that has happened to me, but it reminds me that I am worthy. It reminds me that I can grieve and thrive simultaneously. That I am so much more than the things that have been done to me. That my light is far brighter than my dark.

## Turning Pain into Passion: Transcending Sexual Trauma Through Yoga

A large portion of my professional roles in higher education settings have entailed giving presentations on sexual trauma. I have intersected with thousands of survivors in the past fifteen years doing this work. There have been some themes that have come up consistently. Many survivors have shared that they were looking for something tangible. Something that allowed them to process the painful experiences and triggers that were arising every single day. Many survivors also shared that they did not feel comfortable accessing talk therapy. Due to things like stigma around seeking mental health services and cultural barriers, it is critical we increase accessibility and create different entry points for survivors to seek support.

I knew I wanted to develop a soulful program that spoke to the language of the body. Something that allowed survivors to truly be seen for their diverse identities and experiences. Transcending Sexual Trauma Through Yoga started as a small vision and has now grown in ways beyond my imagination. I am now working with over twenty college campuses and trauma agencies to help them infuse trauma-informed yoga into the scope of their work with survivors, training yoga teachers and mental health professionals across the world in teaching from a trauma-informed lens, and teaching yoga to survivors in a variety of different settings. I am continually amazed and humbled by this work.

My practice has taught me how to be vulnerable and put myself out there despite all the ways trauma makes it easy to feel small. As a woman of color and a survivor, it has taken me years to truly see myself and believe that my voice matters.

## Reminders to Rest in Healing

I'll be honest, it's really challenging for me to rest. To truly rest. I've always been acutely aware that overworking is one of my coping strategies. I'm not sure that I've experienced true, deep rest in a long, long time. For me, trauma compounds this feeling. When responsibilities are endless, it can be impossible to find ways to let go of the feeling of needing to do. To be present with what's in front of me. To turn down the mental chatter and the urgency of the needs of others. To release the guilt that comes with saying no. Some days the anxiety feels like the most overwhelming visceral emotion that swirls around in my gut. It takes over. Like my nervous system has completely collapsed.

Self-care for me is about accessing our internal resources. It is about taking embodiment breaks. Creating transitions in our workday. Taking a mindful approach to our relationships and identifying the ones that no longer serve us. It is prioritizing our time and who and what is worthy of it. It is engaging in activities that nourish and support our nervous systems. When we can be gentle with ourselves and give ourselves permission to ask for what we need, it can be our most powerful resource in recovery.

My practice has taught me that self-care is not a luxury, but rather it is integral to my survival and the ability for everyone I love to also thrive.

And what I know for sure is that the first step to reinforcing our self-worth on a daily basis is recognizing each day that we are worthy of our own love. Like anything else, it is a practice, and not a linear one. It takes all that we have to continue coming back to ourselves, to reevaluate our current practices and identify what needs to change, where we need better boundaries, and when we need to ask for help. It is digging deep and listening to the internal voice that has the answers. We just have to listen. There is such beauty in remembering that we are enough, exactly as we are.

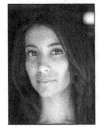

Zabie Yamasaki did her undergraduate in psychology and social behavior at UC Irvine and her graduate in higher education administration at The George Washington University. Zabie is a yoga instructor and has a passion for teaching trauma-informed yoga and training yoga teachers in trauma-informed care. She's the program director of Trauma Informed Programs at UCLA and the founder of Transcending Sexual Trauma Through Yoga. She has been featured on CNN, NBC, and the Huffington Post. You can learn more about her work at zabieyamasaki.com.

Author photo by Garrett Yamasaki.

# BEYOND THE MAT: A PRACTICE FOR COLLECTIVE HEALING

## *Alli Simon*

More than anything, when I look back on my journey, I think about how much I've lost. Some of my earliest life experiences revolve around the loss of a loved one, community, or anything that felt seemingly normal to me. What I remember most are my attempts to find strength and belonging in the midst of those devastating moments.

Although I experienced loss after loss, I don't remember having tools to help me cope with them. There was no therapy, grief counseling, or any active listening. There was nothing more, except learning to get by and make do. I'm 100 percent certain that I wasn't the only person who had this sort of lived experience. Many people in the community I come from are living in a world where they are experts at learning the hard way, navigating a society without equitable wages, and living in neighborhoods that lack basic necessities; therefore, a lot of emotional things that come up are swept under the rug to be dealt with later. The conversation around healing and mental health becomes indefinitely postponed.

Since conversations about healing weren't happening, we definitely weren't practicing yoga or meditation. Even though Los Angeles has one of the largest growing yoga communities in the world, the part of LA that I come from, South LA (particularly South Central which is an area of South LA), is typically excluded from the wellness conversation. Many people still think yoga is a fitness regime that requires Cirque de Soleil-esque flexibility and is something that only "skinny white girls" from the Westside practice. There's also a high chance that someone from my area will tell you that yoga isn't something that people in communities like ours do. Because it isn't for us; it's for them!

"Them"—those are the people who are different than us, evidenced by the way our communities are divided by race and class. "Them" are usually the people who—unlike us—have easier access to things that we don't. They eat kale and quinoa, drive fuel-efficient cars, and rarely travel south of the 10 Freeway. "Them" believe that if we want "healthy" foods, we should abandon our food desert neighborhoods and invest in theirs or wait until ours become "saved" by gentrification. "Them" don't realize that their communities have an abundance of wellness options while ours have very little.

Coupled with limited options, there is an overwhelming stigma that perpetuates the idea that therapy is for the "crazy." Our elders give us the advice, "Be strong," "Don't cry," and "Therapy is for them, not you." Still, with so many barriers, the people of South LA are resilient, with an unmatched strength, and my life is the result of generations who have made unimaginable sacrifices. This story is for US.

## My LA Story

I'm a fifth generation South LA native; my mother was born here as were my grandparents and my great-grandparents. From what I was told, our ancestors migrated long before the first Black migration, which was halfway through the twentieth century. My mother often talks about growing up and LA being such a different place. There was a sense of safety, there were vibrant Black businesses, and overall it was like living in a little village because families were connected and knew one another.

She gave birth to my brother when she was a teen and as a result dropped out of high school. Without an education, she would experience more hardship, but nevertheless, she managed to make things work, not only for myself and my two siblings, but for our extended family and neighbors. As the policies of the '80s and '90s began to transform our South LA home into a literal "war on drugs," people were afraid, and I still look back and remember feeling fearful. I still remember on nights when there was heavy gang activity my siblings and I would get on the floor or huddle under the bathroom sink in case of stray bullets. To this day, the sound of police helicopters reminds me of those traumatic times, as they would often fly over our house shining their invasive lights through our windows day and night.

In spite of those experiences, my mother ensured that we knew there was life outside of what our community could offer us. Most parents in our neighborhood couldn't manage to do this for their kids, but somehow mine did. I'll never forget the time my single mother piled our neighborhood friends and cousins in the car and took us to Disneyland. At the time, I was unaware of the impact these experiences would have on my life, but I do recall them being special.

It was in 1991 when I experienced my first loss. My stepfather was murdered a month after his release from prison. From his death, and the harsh reality that our community was facing, came another loss: our home. In the blink of an eye, we packed up our things and left our family home because my mother couldn't tolerate the pain and the growing tensions in LA any longer.

We spent the next ten years living in a rural part of California. I felt different, I felt alone, and it took years for me to feel like I belonged there. I stuck out like a sore thumb as I was often the only Black kid in my classes. Frankly, I didn't realize this was a "thing" until one of my peers brought it to my attention. One day a classmate used lunchtime to pass around invitations for her birthday party. All of my classmates received an invitation, yet when she got to me, she stopped, then sadly admitted that her father wouldn't allow me to attend because I was Black.

By the time I turned seventeen, I had already attended more than eight funerals. Including my own biological father. Although he was very present in my life, after his death, I don't remember there being conversations about him. I swept him, the feelings around his death, and my emotions under the rug and kept living. Once I finished high school, I moved back to LA. I settled in an area of LA that more closely reflected the quality of life I wished to have, while my mom moved back to South LA. For the first time, as an adult, I became aware of how racial and geographic divides placed barriers on accessing healthy foods, optimal health care, and wellness spaces.

I spent much of my twenties traveling, thanks to my sister who encouraged me to get out of my comfort zone and see the world. I took my first trip abroad to India. It was there that I learned of the divided caste system that places a systemic barrier between people who are born into different social classes. It was also there that I was introduced to OM, the sacred symbol and mantra in the Hindu and Buddhist cultures that represents a universal connection to God. Two contrasting realities, one of societal separation and the other of collective devotion made me cognizant of just how much traveling could help build an understanding of complex social barriers that keep humans disconnected and how spirituality could potentially bring us closer together.

A few years later, I embarked on a six-month study abroad trip to England. Ironically, It was there that I was first introduced to Buddhist meditation practices. My untrained mind initially resisted sitting in silence, but after a few consistent weeks, my mind settled into the practice. Within these solitary moments, I began to feel less "different" and more connected to the world around me. I realized that regardless of where I was, I could feel like home anyplace my feet landed. Home was within me.

On a trip to Costa Rica, I unearthed my connection to yoga—and I hated it! I practiced several times while there and I hid in the very back of the class. The back was a place where both my fatness and Blackness could skip the gaze of white girls traveling to experience "Pura Vida." I never saw anyone who looked like me practicing yoga, so I clung to the assumptions of my community: yoga is only for "them."

Traveling through all of these cities made me present to the divide that happens within ourselves, which is a reflection of the divide that happens within our communities. My world opened up and I began seeing that I was not separate from any one place. Where I was, there I was. I saw that divisions could be erased and communities could be unified through healing.

## Toward Yoga

One week after my trip to Costa Rica, I was struck with yet another loss—my sister. She died in a car accident. This time, loss was different. I was seeing a therapist and had already begun working on healing my old traumas. So when it happened, I couldn't stuff it under like I was able to do growing up. In fact, everything in my life completely stopped.

Things quickly became consumed by loss. My best friend contracted HIV and began fighting for his life, a battle I was present for that he eventually lost. My ten-year-old beagle died of cancer, and I lost my job after being forced to choose between being with my family or climbing the corporate nonprofit ladder. Within the span of a year, my life became unrecognizable, and I felt like I had nothing except my ability to quiet my mind.

I needed to make some immediate changes before I had a mental breakdown. I'd stopped practicing asana (poses) but I continued to meditate, often three times a day. Meditation was less about functioning in my world or about escaping my sadness. I needed meditation to figure out what was next for me. I found myself searching for meaning everywhere. What was the meaning of it all? Who was I? WHY was all of this happening to me? I had entered my own personal hell.

I visited a doctor who prescribed me medications for anxiety. Me? Anxious? No, thank you! I declined pharmaceuticals not because I didn't think they would help but because I carried the stigma that taking medication would mean I was "crazy"—so I requested that we try holistic methods. She recommended that I return to the physical practice of yoga.

## Toward Liberation

Yoga. The practice I hated because of my chubby body, lack of flexibility, and dismal upper body strength was no longer a match for the amount of pain I felt. I began to practice daily. Almost immediately, I began to understand just how precious each BREATH I took was, and each time I closed my eyes and connected to my heart, I knew my life had meaning.

I found a yoga studio that offered group classes a block from my home. I saw my therapist weekly. I committed to and used yoga as my healing. I didn't care that my body was curvy or how my hips were bigger than every person in the room. I needed something to get my mind off of the sadness and grief I was experiencing. The more I practiced, the more I loved it. Not because it was perfect or helped me to forget but because with each posture, it proved that I was capable of more than I ever thought was possible.

One day, while in pigeon, I felt my breath move throughout my entire body, and my hips opened wider, causing me to fall deeper into it. I burst into tears, right there on my mat. Every moment of my life had brought me to this point. I instinctively knew that all of my experiences were shaped in order to bring my heart, body, and mind to this mat.

Coming to my mat urged me to look at my body in a different way. It became a metaphor for vulnerability and inspired me to open myself up while off the mat too. I witnessed how yoga could be used as a backdoor to healing. Not just for "them" but for people like *me*.

I no longer wanted to hide in the back of the class. I wanted people to see me—in all my Blackness and fatness—front and center of the class. I wanted to shift my community's shared idea of who practiced yoga. I wanted them to see that people like me could practice yoga and be from South LA. We are multifaceted and I wanted everyone to know.

## Sharing the Practice

It became clear to me that I was being called to share yoga and meditation with the community that I called home. I shunned the idea of running away to "safer" or more beautiful communities, as these areas are already saturated with yoga studios. I moved back home to South LA and devoted my practice to sharing yoga in spaces with those who look like me, who were still battling their own misconceptions of healing.

I committed to making this practice accessible for everyone. Everyone included people of color, young people, elders, queer and trans people, those with curvy bodies, and anyone who felt left out in the trendy Western style of yoga and meditation that LA is known for. I began developing yoga and meditation techniques that aimed to remind students of yoga of this truth: that yoga is for everyone. Moving away from culturally appropriated practices that are harmful, I've found ways to make my practice more relatable to my community. On Tuesday, you'll find me playing my Solange or Miles Davis playlist while helping an elder with a posture variation. On Sundays, my class enjoys some old Radiohead while I demonstrate how queer and larger-bodied folx should and can take up space. And each day, I am prioritizing consent and reminding the class that they are their own teacher and I am just their guide.

Lately, I am envisioning what a world could look like for people who are silently suffering from grief, the results of violence, mass incarceration, depression, and marginalization. If they were offered access to something else that looked accessible and familiar, what could be achieved?

My story isn't about how we can teach people to eat better, meditate their pain away, and "asana" the strength to endure their trauma. Instead, I offer this practice as an invitation to recognize that there is the possibility of resilience. There is rich history in communities that are often left out of the conversation of yoga and meditation. At the same time there are systemic and unethical realities that place a barrier between people and healing.

In my practice today, I close with an expression of gratitude and a reminder that each student is their own teacher and that their practice is for them, not for anyone else. We focus on breath with the intention of bringing these tools to their world beyond the mat. Change isn't done alone; it's achieved through a collective effort, it's incremental, and it's a slow process.

Although conversations around mental wellness and healing have been historically swept under the rug, having access to contemplative practices like yoga and meditation can be a pathway to personal and collective liberation. As it has done for me, this work can inspire folks to stand up against systems of injustice that create barriers, because healing and self-care isn't just for "THEM" and their communities and their bodies but also for US, our communities, and our bodies.

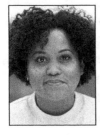

Alli Simon (she/her) is a South LA native, 200-hour certified yoga and meditation facilitator. She commits her energy to working with nonprofits dedicated to systems change, workplace wellness, and healing justice. She believes in increasing access to self-care practices like meditation, yoga, and therapy for marginalized people to help foster a more resilient and loving world. For more, visit www.allisimon.com.

Author photo by Emily Knecht.

# SAMSKARA, GRIEF, TRAUMA, AND JOY

## *Kathryn Templeton*

At one point in my young life, I wanted to be a public defender. In my first criminal law class, my professor asked the question, "Are fairness and justice the same thing?" I raised my hand high, almost bouncing with excitement about my slam dunk answer. After stating my argument as to why I believed, with my whole twenty-one-year-old heart, that they were the same thing, I was asked to come to the front of the classroom. My professor slowly and deliberately spoke to me, for all to hear, in his deep Southern drawl, "My dear Kathryn, you are going to be the saddest lawyer in the land! Take yourself across the quad to social work school. That is where the belief that fairness and justice stand side by side, not in the American court system."

This was a hard and humbling moment, for which I am eternally grateful. I have since made a career out of working with the human heart, mind, and soul, living in a world where fairness and justice are not always at the same table.

My work is in grief, trauma, and joy. While these may not seem a likely threesome, they are in fact deeply interwoven, and together they create a net, catching moments in our lives that inform how we see the world. As a trauma therapist, it is critical for me to be able to model vulnerability and to be versed in working with grief of the heart, confusion of the mind, and feelings of disconnection from meaning and spirit.

My stories reflect these narratives. Memory is key in all of these tales. From my father's slow whittling away, his great intellect shaved off piece by piece from dementia, to one of my more memorable clients, whose family history repeated patterns of behavior creating generations of pain.

My professor was right: fairness and justice are not the same and neither are memory and reality. The relationship is dependent, in both cases, on the belief of the individual.

## Part I: Losing My Mind

My dad and I were taking a walk just before sunset one day in 1999. He was six foot six inches tall, and I sufficiently less tall. His stride was so long, I had to take two steps to meet his one. I recalled when I was a little girl walking with my dad, just before sunset, and taking two skips with my arm reaching up high to hold my father's hand. We both loved these walks, for very different reasons I'm sure, yet they were something that we could both count on to lift us up.

In 1999, Dad had advanced Alzheimer's disease (AD). He and I would take our walk and he would say to me, "I know I love you honey ... I just don't know your name." We would laugh and smile at each other.

I would say to him, "That's okay Dad, all the sailors say that to me, no worries." Again, we would laugh.

That is how Alzheimer's disease can operate; the affect or feeling is still there, but the ability to put the words to it is diminished or erased. Watching my dad deconstruct was heartbreaking.

I had worked at the Institute on Aging in San Francisco as an intern in the Alzheimer's Disease Unit in graduate school. The disease had been my focus in my post-graduate work, and when my dad finally had all other potential illnesses ruled out, we both knew it was AD. Dad had read up on dementia. He was a brilliant, NYT-crossword-puzzle-with-pen kinda guy.

Our walks had always been our connection time, and between 1992 and 2001, he would share with me what it was like to "lose his mind." Dad told me that his mind was like sand: holding that sand in his hands, he could sense his memories were simply falling between his fingers, unable to be caught.

We were all there when he died. I had stayed the night in his hospice room and tried to match his breathing pattern. This was something I had learned when working at the AIDS Hospice in the 1980s, another internship back in grad school. We were taught that when someone is dying they will often breathe in a manner called "chain stoking," with long pauses in between inhale and exhale. This is a difficult pattern to match and attempting to often brings up emotions. Yet breathing with someone is an intimate mirror, and the theory was that if someone is unconscious, they may feel supported by having their breath mirrored back to them. It was all we had in common at that moment. It was how I could stride with Dad as he died. Two steps to his one, trying to stay ahold of his hand.

After Dad died, I became completely obsessed with breath. I began to search for information on breathing techniques. I found them in yoga. I started with breathing practices, then *asana* (poses), and finally meditation.

My studies with breathing practices and yoga led me to study ayurveda (the medical branch of the spiritual practices of yoga). I was struck by the similarities between Western psychology and ayurvedic medicine. I used these tools in my work at an urban public health clinic where I worked with many families and children who were diagnosed with Complex Trauma (C-PTSD).[12]

Working in the field of clinical psychotherapy has offered many rewards. I am in awe of the vulnerability and the courage of clients to address the experiences in their lives.

12. Complex PTSD, defined in 1988 by Dr. Judith Herman of Harvard University, is intended to "describe the symptoms of long-term trauma." The following symptoms are part of her formulation: somatization, interpersonal difficulties, cognitive difficulties, emotional difficulties, and behavioral difficulties. "Complex PTSTD" PTSD: National Center for PTSD, US Department of Veterans Affairs, accessed March 4, 2020, https://www.ptsd.va.gov/professional/treat/essentials/complex_ptsd.asp.

## Part II: Samskara (History Repeats Itself)

One such client was a seventeen-year-old girl I'll refer to as "Tisha" who had been a client at the clinic for over ten years. During that time, she had seen several therapists. We were a teaching clinic, and that means that once a student's internship was complete, the client would be moved to a new therapist. Sometimes, as was the case when I worked with Tisha, the clients would be with a full-time clinical specialist, but after a while there was generally some shift in caseloads. This is an important detail to note, as building relationship, trust, and communication is often a challenge for our C-PTSD clients, as it is for so many of us.

Tisha and I met for a number of sessions due to her report of a recent episode of sexual assault. This was not the first sexual assault that Tisha had experienced. However, this time was different, as she reported, "I was raped, got pregnant, and decided to abort the baby." She went on to report, "Everyone is mad at me for the abortion. Nobody seems to care how it all happened."

Tisha had a diagnosis that made her vulnerable to victimization and a family with a vast trauma history: multiple recent deaths, violence, and extreme poverty. However, it was not until I met her mother and grandmother that I realized how deep the samskaras around sexual assault were imprinted from an epigenetic standpoint.

Epigenetic medicine is an intersection between Western and Eastern medicine. The ayurvedic idea of samskaras and the science of epigenetics are closely related. According to ayurveda, physical, emotional, and behavioral imprints (called *samskaras*) are carried from generation to generation. In Western medicine, these imprints are called linked neural pathways. (A neural pathway is created from repetition of behavior over time, or the intensity of a behavior or event.)

## Impressions Are Like Ghosts in the Mind

A samskara, as defined by Pandit Rajmani Tigunait, PhD, the spiritual head of the Himalayan Institute, is "'the impression of, the impact of, the action we perform with full awareness of its goals.' When we perform such an action, a subtle impression is deposited in our mindfield.

Each time the action is repeated, the impression becomes stronger. This is how a habit is formed."[13]

In our session with Tisha's mother and grandmother it was disclosed that Tisha was the "baby of a rape," as her mother shared that she herself was assaulted when she was sixteen years old. Tisha's grandmother reported that "T's Mom [Tisha's mother] was conceived when [I was] seventeen and raped by a man who lived in my neighborhood."

I had called Tisha's mom and grandmother into session, as Tisha was reporting she was being "shamed about the rape." There was now more understanding about how Tisha's sexual assault triggered her family, and they came to session to talk about their mixed feelings around Tisha's "breaking out" from the family pattern by choosing not to have her baby.

These types of habitual actions are not always activated. In fact, there is the ability to change the samskara or repair multigenerational patterns by becoming conscious of them. These imprints do not have to be carried to offspring; rather, by bringing the unconscious into conscious awareness, they can be altered, and new behaviors or associations can be installed, thus creating change in tendency and behavior.

Tisha's case is an extreme example of samskara. We can more easily identify biological samskaras such as alcoholism, sickle cell anemia, or depression. Behavioral tendencies are also examples of unconscious experiences, that have been passed down through generations of DNA, with years of habitual actions in ancestral diet, environmental factors, and cultural traumas. Not all samskaras are problems; in fact, many are healthy and useful. For example, our inherent immunity to various diseases is from our DNA and RNA and behavioral tendencies.

I watched when Jack, my middle son, then six years old, put one hand on his hip and the other behind his head and swiveled his hips. This was something that my dad would do when he wanted to break the tension in the room. He called it his "Big Jay Hula dance." Jack had never seen my father do this, as Dad died when Jack was only four years

---

13. Pandit Rajmani Tigunait, "What Are Samskaras and How Do They Affect Us?" Yoga International, accessed February 24, 2020, https://yogainternational.com /article/view/what-are-samskaras-and-how-do-they-affect-us.

old. My dad was deep in the throes of AD when Jack was born. Yet there it was, my father's hula dance being performed by my six-year-old son in the cafeteria of his elementary school. The principal gave me a call telling me that Jack had been doing his "Barbie dance" whenever he got nervous because someone was getting into trouble—in the cafeteria, classroom, and in the gym. While she agreed it was "hard not to laugh, as his performance was hysterical," it was creating a distraction that was hard for the teachers and staff to manage. Dad's coping mechanism of silly dance, his tendency to create a humorous distraction to decrease tension, was deeply embedded in Jack's DNA.

This idea of samskara can also be another lens through which to view tendencies toward alcoholism, depression, and anxiety. While my brother and I both share the same DNA, he has been the only one to have squamous cell cancer, degenerative spinal issues, and GI issues. Why? Epigenetics might suggest, as would yoga science and ayurveda, that although these imprints are present in both of us, whether or not they become activated could vary due to our consciousness and attention to choosing different habitual actions.

In ayurveda we have a *dinacharya*, or daily routine, that offers us gentle cleansing and rejuvenation with simple behaviors: tongue scraping, drinking water in the morning, waking up with the sun, practicing simple asana and meditation. This type of daily action (repetition and time) sets up a new imprint. This has been my practice for almost twenty years now.

My brother did not have access to this information, and ever since he was in the Vietnam War, he has smoked cigarettes. He has also made a habit of drinking six Coca-Colas a day and practices unconscious eating patterns. You could argue that these regular habits, along with the multiple traumas he experienced while being a navy medic in the war, conspired to epigenetically open up samskaras in his mind that might be lying dormant in my own DNA.

Personal responsibility is important in our health and well-being. Having access to the science of yoga and ayurveda is helpful. Yet the most important aspect of changing samskaras is creating awareness where there once was none. This means becoming conscious and making decisions based upon your internal locus of control—your "inner voice"—versus the habitual voice of our unconscious society (i.e., an *external* locus of control).

## Just Listen

How do I know this? Because, like you, I have been through stuff and found my way out of the many tunnels of grief that follow loss. The boat that has carried me along these grief-canals has been my yoga practice. The community, or *sangha*, that surrounds me due to that practice, and the ability to be comfortable with myself—to give myself time and space to grieve—are all byproducts of yoga, at least in my experience.

There is another river that feeds into my grief-canal, and that is my professional work as a trauma therapist. Over twenty-five years of sitting with children, teenagers, and adults, listening to them share their narratives. Just listening and sometimes offering tea. My work led me to yoga, to ayurveda, and eventually back home to myself.

My father's voice is in my mind reminding me to appreciate every day. To try to allow the moments of joy to be recorded in my mind, my heart, and in the shared experiences with my family and friends that mark the seasons.

These collective experiences help us hold ourselves together. We see and experience ourselves as a member of a tribe, a group, a pack. If I had not allowed myself to grieve for my father, to feel the horrible heartbreak of loss, I would not have his perspective to hold me, to appreciate my memory, all of my memories. Not to hold on to them by gripping but to allow myself to carefully select the memories that inform how I view my life now.

Clients like Tisha, and movements like Jack's "Big Jay Hula/Barbie dance" remind me that my tendencies are not just mine alone. I share many attributes with my ancestors, and I carry the family DNA into each of my waking breaths. The more I try to meditate, become more conscious, and actively take responsibility for choices that guide and direct my life, the more I replace unhealthy samskaras with healthier ones and offer myself a greater sense of freedom in my life. None of this is done without effort. Choosing to see clearly with the eyes of conscious awareness does not always win me friends or conform to what is hip. Yet at the end of the day I sleep well. I rise with the sun and can tolerate the waves of life with less stress and greater appreciation for the voyage. My mind may too become like sand, spilling out from between my fingers. But for now I am wholehearted, with my mind and heart connected and a deep gratitude for being able to listen and sometimes offer tea.

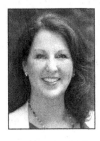

Kathryn Templeton, MA, LPC, C-IAYT, E500RYT, ayurveda practitioner, has devoted her life to the health of others. A psychotherapist for thirty years working clinically in the treatment of anxiety, depression, and complex trauma, Kathryn has developed protocols integrating the principles of yoga therapy, ayurvedic medicine, and psychology. Kathryn is a faculty member at the Himalayan Institute where she is the director of Himalayan Institute Ayurvedic Programs. She is the founder of 3WT- Wellness Coach Program with Yoga International.

Author photo by Andrea Killam.

# PART THREE: REFLECTION QUESTIONS

- What occurs within me when I lean into the natural cycle of birth and death?
- What do I notice when I acknowledge the full range of emotions I experience in any given moment?
- What lessons have I learned from my experience of grief and loss?
- How has my experience of grief and loss connected me to the suffering others experience?
- What practices do I employ to heal myself in the midst of grieving?

—Michelle C. Johnson

# PART FOUR

## *Exploring the Intersection of Trauma and Identity*

Each one of us holds multiple identities whether we're aware of them or not. Each one of us has a gender identity and sexual orientation, a race and ethnicity, a socioeconomic status or class, an age, a size, a religious affiliation or sense of spirituality (or not, an identity in and of itself), as well as being marked by certain physical abilities or (invisible and visible) disabilities.

These aggregated and overlapping identities impact our experience of ourselves, one another, the world at large and, in turn, how others and the larger society experience and interact with us. This is true whether we're aware of it or not, whether we like it or not. Some of us are more aware than others, as certain individuals may experience identities classified as the "dominant" group affording certain privileges or opportunities, including not having to take stock of or experience these identities on a day-to-day basis. Other individuals may have fewer identities associated with the dominant group and more identities that are classified as "marginalized," often referred to as "minority groups."

When it comes to trauma, the source and experience of our traumas intersects with the complexities of our identities and the places we occupy in the social structure as a result of those identities. This is also true when it comes to our access to and experience of healing modalities.

In "Nonrecognition and Healing Transgender Trauma with Yoga," Tobias Wiggins shares the ways in which gender binaries in yoga environments often unintentionally create unsafe spaces. He examines a series of events and interactions which reenact and affirm the transphobic and exclusionary space of mainstream culture and explains how these normalized, and invisible conventions may lead to even further trauma. Wiggins then shares and outlines a new vision of how yoga, specifically trauma-informed yoga, can heal and not further harm.

Many people assume body image and body acceptance "challenges" are reserved for cisgender women. That holds true in the yoga world where stereotypes of lithe, able "yoga bodies" dominate social media and most yoga imagery from print ads to magazine covers. In "My Buddha Body," Michael Hayes breaks down these assumptions while discussing his own experience as a large-bodied black man and yoga teacher. He provides the reader an opportunity to examine how race, size, and gender, as held or projected identities, interact with tropes about the normalized and fetishized "yoga body." He not only shares his journey to determine how his actions define him but offers questions for us to reflect on how we interact with ourselves and one another.

In "From Vicious Cycles to Virtuous Cycles: Healing Childhood Sexual Trauma," Susanna Barkataki details her journey from disassociation to reclamation through yoga and mindfulness practices. As a "body-based practice," yoga allowed Susanna to reconnect and establish a healthy relationship to her body and her culture of origin by working from the inside out. This gift of liberation ignited her to share the ways in which not only she, but others, can experience healing and transformation. As Barkataki powerfully states, "As more of us become aware of this system and change it, we even prevent the trauma from occurring in the first place."

Amber Karnes reclaims the word "fat" and her body in "Yoga Turned My Body into a Place I Could Call Home." Explicitly and implicitly told that her fat body was her primary identity and that it was not valued, yoga offered her the space to truly be in her body. It offered her an embodied experience of self as well as peace, something she now leads others to experience—unapologetically and completely.

Rachel Otis explores the various parts of her identity and her efforts to integrate and disintegrate, demonstrating the complex and layered nature of our sense of self in "Somewhere Under the Rainbow." From race and ethnicity, to religion and national origin, to gender identity and sexual orientation, to size and dis/ability, Rachel outlines the intersectional nature of not only her identity but her way of being and experiencing the world (and how the world has responded in turn). From internalizing hatred and waging war on her body, Rachel recounts her journey into wholeness, self-acceptance, and the depth and breadth of body positivity as not only a slogan but a mission.

In "My Own Hero: Healing My Inner Black Gay Child," Dorian Christian Baucum paints a vivid picture of his past, one in which his neighborhood, socioeconomic status, the time period in which he grew up, and the expectations of his sex all aggressively and often violently intersected with his sexual orientation and expression of "masculinity." Neither were acceptable and received vehement and frequent reminders that there was something "wrong" with him. In fact, simply being himself was considered a betrayal by many of the men in his world. Through creative expression and yoga, he recounts his journey into healing and wholeness.

Niralli Tara D'Costa rounds out this section with "Movement of Awakening" in which she focuses on the various movement practices she's explored and added to her repertoire of healing over the years. Like puzzle pieces or steps on a perfectly aligned pathway, each modality offered new possibilities and opportunities for her to be present and fully embodied as she experienced healing and growth. At the root, her capacity for these practices all stem from the daily fiber of yoga and meditation in her life as an Indian woman.

# MEDITATION

## *Deep Love*

During this practice you are going to connect with your deep capacity to love yourself. You may not feel like loving yourself right now, and this is a practice and invitation to begin to allow self-love to find a place in your heart. This is a practice that invites you to fall in love with yourself.

We will start with a breathing practice to quiet your mind.

Find a comfortable seat or, if you prefer, you can stand or lie down. To find a comfortable seat, you might want to elevate your hips by sitting on a cushion, pillow, or blanket.

Close your eyes or look at the ground in front of you and begin to breathe into your body. Start by taking deep breaths in and out. Begin to feel the shape change in your body as you breathe.

Notice the physical sensations and the emotions.

Now, bring your awareness to your heart, the space where your heart lives.

Breathe into the heart for a few cycles of breath.

As you breathe, ask yourself what story or narrative is blocking you from loving yourself. Often narratives come from culture, family, or something outside of us. For example: I'm not good enough. I'm unlovable. I don't belong.

Once you've identified the story or narrative that is blocking you from loving yourself, invite it to be released, even if just for one cycle of breath. Invite it to release from your heart and spirit. You can invite it to be released by breathing it out of your body with your exhales and making space for something new to enter as you inhale.

Work this way for several cycles of breath, emphasizing your exhales and release.

Now come back to your heart, the space where your heart lives. Notice how your heart feels. Notice what is present and if possible, create a mantra about self-love. This can be something you already believe or something you want to believe. For example: I am enough! I am loveable! I belong here! or I have a place here!

Repeat your mantra three times.

Once you feel ready to move out of meditation, with each breath cycle bring your awareness back to the physical sensations and emotions. Return to the space by opening your eyes.

—Michelle C. Johnson

# NONRECOGNITION AND HEALING TRANSGENDER TRAUMA WITH YOGA

## Tobias Wiggins

This space is dark, humid, and peaceful. Polished hardwood floors have been packed mat to mat with those seeking assorted reliefs. It's one refuge from the city's reliable turbulence, which has now been reduced to a dim chatter outside the window, opaque with condensation from our collective exertion. I realize that, although muted by the studio walls, I can hear the noise clearer now. In moments like these I'm reminded that the effort of finding presence is a subtle bed upon which to lie—not always comfortable or memorable but ultimately prepared for the weight of your body and its story.

Like most contemporary yoga studios, I can tell that the creation of a safer space is a priority here. Poses are fine-tuned, teachers are well acquainted with physiology and various contraindications. They offer considerate adaptations for all levels of practice and body types. They remind us not to push ourselves too far and often share tips for self-care, sometimes laced with philosophy, mythology, or the teacher's personal insights. The baseboards are lined with fire-safe LED candle replicants, an emulation of flame that accentuates how, in a Western context, safety often blurs with liability. So today, I find myself here, in an eclectic healing environment that could be any urban yoga studio.

The instructor is leading the class through guided meditation about the way energy, information, and matter move through tangible entrances to the body. She shares that this practice should help us foster intention around what we "take in" and what we "give out." Floating around the room, her voice falls gently on our stillness as we rest in savasana: "...there are nine or ten anatomical gates...like doors swinging on hinges. These doors can be well oiled or not." Her voice melodic and catching. "This is where the inside becomes outside and the outside in...there are two eyes, two ears...two nostrils...one mouth, one anus..." She takes a pregnant pause before naming the genitals. I know her words are genuine, yet they suddenly feel unduly sanguine, so sweet my tongue turns sticky and I am overly aware of it in my mouth. My panic vibrates with anticipation of what she is about to do—my muscles tense, mind dissociates, breathing shallows, and time slows while speeding up. When she arrives at the final openings, she explains that men have one doorway whereas women have two.

For most cisgender[14] people, this final gendered bodily statement may seem obvious, unremarkable, or even progressive in its lack of corporeal shame and a decentering of males as the default.[15] However, for people whose gender has changed from the one they were assigned at birth (such as those who are transgender,[16] two-spirit, non-binary, or agender) or for intersex people, this simple equation of gender to genital configuration may not only be inaccurate (not all women have vaginas, for example) but also quite harmful. And particularly within the vulnerability and unguardedness that can be elicited by a somatic heal-

14. "Cisgender" means those who identify with the gender they were assigned at birth.

15. The assertion that some people have ten gates is actually a subversion of the traditional way of conceptualizing the entrances to the body, which would default to the masculine and assert that everyone has only nine openings.

16. Throughout the remainder of this chapter, I use transgender and trans as umbrella terms, which encompass but are not limited to identifications including two-spirit, non-binary, transsexual, genderqueer, gender non-conforming, MTF, FTM, transwoman, transman, bi-gendered, and agender. It should be noted that not all those listed under this umbrella may identify as "transgender."

ing practice like yoga, such an oversight could even, in itself, be experienced as acutely traumatizing.

This recounting[17] is only one segment of a vast collection of episodes that have occurred during my many years of practice at yoga studios. As a transgender person, I am aware that entering any cisgender-dominated space surely means a confrontation with systemic transphobia. And to be clear I'm not talking about the kind of transphobia that manifests by active exclusion, like an obvious expression of hatred or violence—prejudiced attributes from which most liberal thinkers exempt themselves.

Rather, the transphobia I encounter in most healing venues is subtler and more consistent, a collection of normalized, often well-meaning behaviors, which could also be called microaggressions. These are harmful conventions made invisible through being so commonplace. And since they slip under the radar, they are easily reproduced or explained away. Some additional examples that are yoga-specific include binary gender bathrooms, registration forms, and change areas; cueing that reduces men's and women's bodies to physical stereotypes or draws on gendered bodily assumptions; the uncritical use of gendered yoga philosophy; a major shortage of transgender representation in students and teachers; and a general lack of understanding regarding how to create a safer space for transgender students, such as proper pronoun use.

Because these systemic issues and behaviors are denied, I am often left carrying the weight of a painful nonrecognition. This nonrecognition stretches beyond my own personal experiences of transphobia to every moment I see that one of my trans peers may be unintentionally cast outside a therapeutic space or may avoid them altogether for fear of such an encounter. It is not only that cisgender people have difficulty envisioning what it means to create an authentic environment that includes transgender yoga practitioners. Beyond inclusion, yoga classes and therapies will only successfully facilitate healing for marginalized communities when they de-privilege cisgender people—as well as

---

17. The specific details of this event have been altered for anonymity and are based upon several overlapping experiences of transphobia at yoga studios. They do not refer to any particular individual or business.

white, straight, able-bodied, middle-class, thin settlers—as the accepted norm.

The following chapter moves to discuss how creating a trauma-informed yoga space requires knowledge and understanding of the "everydayness" of this systemic oppression. I will underscore the ways that somatic therapy can effectively address many trans-specific psychological and physical difficulties—difficulties that are often ignored or left untreated from medical doctors and in mainstream health care. However, yoga can only truly be a healing tool for transgender populations if the larger yoga community actively addresses the centering of privileged identities and the covert exclusion of marginalized people. I therefore end by discussing a new vision for trauma-informed practice, one which offers practical solutions for challenging transphobia in studios and teaching.

## Everyday Trauma

Author and psychotherapist Mark Epstein discusses the quotidian nature of trauma, explaining that, especially in our contemporary world, it is difficult to live without being exposed to an event that overtakes our protective mental, spiritual, or physical faculties.[18] The traumatic moment is simply one which we cannot metabolize. It is an event so overwhelming to our senses that the body struggles to work through it, and in this way, we do not come to fully know what exactly has transpired. It leaves traces of unthought thoughts, subliminal evidence in the ever-present folds of our history. In this way traumatic memories get stored like etchings under the skin, their rough edges often rousing symptoms like some of those I experienced during the "bodily gates" meditation: hyperarousal, dissociative numbing, negative self-image, and somatization.[19]

Marginalized people are those populations who are sidelined and face oppression based upon their identity, appearance, or social difference. For these communities, the "everydayness" of trauma can take

---

18. Mark Epstein, *The Trauma of Everyday Life* (New York: The Penguin Press, 2013), 26.

19. A somatization can be defined as a physical manifestation of psychological distress. This physical symptom may not have a clear organic cause, disappearing only when the underlying psychological issue has been addressed.

on an additional dimension: it holds the distinctive impact of power relations, inflicted by hierarchies that consistently place one group of people above another. For those who are transgender, this materializes in a wide range of potentially injurious occurrences from childhood throughout adult life.

Transgender youth often confront misgendering and nonacceptance at the hands of their primary caregivers, in school, or from peer groups. They may be denied appropriate health care, have their gender identity policed, or have restrictions placed on lifesaving interventions like hormonal therapy. Throughout life, transgender people face continued gatekeeping around health care, the loss or denial of work simply because they are trans, medical pathologization or fetishization, and continued possible rejection from family, friends, or romantic interests. They subsequently encounter disproportionately higher rates of houselessness, mental health struggles like depression, and suicidal ideation. Along with the ever-prevalent de-validation of their personhood, many trans people must vigilantly navigate daily risks of physical and emotional violence. This is especially true for those who have additional marginalizations, such as those who are BIPOC (black, indigenous, people of color), sex workers, and those with disabilities.

I am a white, queer, transgender man who grew up rurally, and as such, there are many aspects of these experiences of harm that I know intimately, while others I have managed to evade through my own privilege and through luck. But regardless of each transgender person's navigation of the unique shape that everyday oppression takes, like most forms of psychological trauma, it often leaves a mark that resides both in the mind and the body.

In any moment that I sense the likelihood for (even well-intentioned) transphobia, like a mistaken pronoun or a probing question about identity, my body jumps into full action. The sympathetic nervous system triggers a cascade of effects to keep me safe—numbing me from ignorant words, preparing for a fight, or initiating my capacity to escape. For a lot of people who are dealing with the symptomatology of PTSD or complex trauma, the body remembers and repeatedly protects against the harmful event, even when there is no present risk. However, for those who are subject to a social world that systemically excludes them, objectifies, tokenizes, disbelieves their identity, or even actively hopes for their extinction, often the real threat has not fully passed.

## Transgender Healing

There is much compelling writing emerging on the power that yoga and meditation can have to help trauma survivors heal by directly addressing what many other therapeutic modalities miss. David Emerson, who founded the Trauma Sensitive Yoga program for the Trauma Center Justice Resource Institute in Massachusetts, elaborates that as an embodied practice, trauma-sensitive yoga functions on multiple interlocking levels. Through a combination of breath, movement, and mindfulness, survivors may use yoga to reconnect to their internal lives, re-instill bodily ownership, facilitate self-acceptance, generate hope for a future, and develop self-soothing skills. Through the emphasis of choice, patience, and interception, these students are potentially able to build new neural pathways through a non-judgmental experience of internal states.[20]

As a person who has faced multiple forms of traumatic injury—including complex childhood trauma, sexual assault, and recurring violence from sexism, homophobia, and transphobia—I have consistently returned to yoga as a form of emotional and spiritual therapy. Granted, for a lot of my life I didn't consciously apprehend what yoga was doing for my mental health. I just found myself recurrently gravitating back to the practice despite serious qualms about the lack of queer and transgender teachers or about the largely unaddressed racism, cultural appropriation, and ableism occurring in Western yoga contexts. Although I often didn't feel entirely safe, reflected, or like the larger yoga community cared to be accountable for the broader social harms they were

20. David Emerson & Elizabeth Hopper, *Overcoming Trauma through Yoga: Reclaiming the Body* (Berkeley, California: North Atlantic Books, 2011), 92-284. This type of trauma-sensitive yoga is a therapeutic intervention and should be differentiated from the type of yoga practiced at the typical studio. That said, many of the techniques and insights garnered from clinical work with those with PTSD and C-PTSD can be used to facilitate a safer, trauma-informed space for clients from a variety of backgrounds.

causing, a part of me knew that through yoga I could touch a kernel of recovery that I wasn't able to find elsewhere.

Many marginalized people therefore practice yoga specifically because it can help manage both psychological and physical stress that is identity specific. For example, transgender people may have an acute feeling of being disconnected from their bodies, whether from gender dysphoria or everyday traumatic experiences.[21] Others have taken up behaviors related to their gender expression or safety, like hiding or exaggerating parts of the body, that can have a mix of positive and negative physical outcomes. Additionally, because of the binary-gender nature of most sports and activities (teams, changerooms), transgender people often have restricted access to the kinship and networks that surround physical recreation.

Before I was able to access surgery, I spent many years wearing a tight compression garment, popularly known as a chest binder. Beyond being an exciting and important tool for my gender expression, this notoriously uncomfortable nylon sleeve not only caused me to chronically tense forward but also severely restricted my breathing—so much so that even in the rare occasion that I was not binding, shallow breath became my involuntary standard. This physicality was so engrained that even after my surgery, for a long time I shouldered the layered, embodied map of years spent fighting for access to the services that allowed me to live.

So like many of those who have histories of trauma, as a matter of psychological survival, I creatively learned how to disconnect from my body on multiple levels. At its simplest, yoga helped me to recognize this separation while also inviting the option of other forms of breath and bodily acceptance. I certainly discovered that my chest could be reopened with asana after its years of collapse, including very practical breathing techniques for regulation and grounding. But perhaps more importantly, over time the practice has taught me unique ways to

---

21. To be clear, although transgender people do have overlapping experiences, there is no uniform transgender life, especially considering a globalized context. Not all transgender people identify with the experience of what is currently called "gender dysphoria," for example.

release all the associated judgments, so I could truly reclaim this formidable history as my own.

As a somatic practice of mind-body awareness, yoga can provide an unparalleled venue for holistic therapeutic healing. It can help transgender practitioners notice relationships between their physical and emotional lives, build new ways of thinking about their body (related to gender or not), fortify self-worth, and facilitate a novel sense of external and internal agency. By stimulating the parasympathetic nervous system in a community-based setting, transgender people who do studio yoga may be able to relax an otherwise unwavering hypervigilance while simultaneously inviting beneficial motion, strength, and flexibility. Yet clearly, these possibilities will only materialize if trans people do not risk re-traumatization by the very spaces that offer refuge.

## A New Vision for Trauma-Informed Practice

At their most optimistic, when instructors discuss trauma and yoga, the ultimate focus falls upon how pursuing asana, meditation, and pranayama can support survivors on their reparative path. A trauma-informed lens goes one step further, facilitating this journey by taking into consideration techniques that avoid unintentionally triggering their students. For example, teachers may cultivate agency through anti-authoritative language when cueing. This includes the avoidance of commands, instead inviting students to try particular movements "if you'd like" or "when you're ready."[22] The use of consent cards has been another way that some studios are trying to shift from a culture of non-consensual touch and adjustments.[23]

Yet, as I have been emphasizing throughout this chapter, developments in trauma-informed yoga have largely failed to mindfully navigate each practitioner's identity and social-political location. I have focused on transgender people's lives; however, all people with a marginalized identity face potential harm through a confrontation with systemic op-

---

22. Emerson, *Trauma-Sensitive Yoga in Therapy*, 9.

23. Tobias Wiggins, "Creating a Culture of Consent through Yoga Practice," Union Yoga + Wellness, August 2, 2017, http://www.unionyogastudio.ca/creating-a-culture-of-consent-through-yoga/.

pression. For example, yoga in the West is enmeshed with histories of colonization and racism.[24] One manifestation of this dynamic is that many yoga studios are run and staffed by majority white people, and the popular image of the contemporary yogi is a white, thin, middle class, cisgender woman. The dominance of Eurocentric whiteness and the violence of cultural appropriation could also be experienced as triggering or re-traumatizing.

Whether in clinical or studio-based work, those who teach yoga will only effectively provide therapeutic interventions if the dynamics of everyday oppression are thoroughly taken into consideration. I believe that if practitioners wish to be comprehensively trauma informed, studios and instructors must first address the impact of invisibilized systems of marginalization like transphobia, and second, they must honor how each person's various intersecting identities can inform their healing, their suffering, and their specific risks of physical or psychological injury during a class.

This larger vision would include transgender-competent yoga classes that address the persistent centering of cisgender people. If I were to dream aloud, I would imagine that all yoga environments (including any forms and websites) transformed to be de-gendered and explicitly welcoming of trans folks, where people can change clothes, shower, and pee safely without fear. Yoga teachers and staff would be thoroughly educated on transgender people's identities and specific needs so they feel like confident, non-defensive allies, who are aware of potential for misgendering, the prevalent use of reductive gender stereotypes, and the complexities of systemic transphobia. Studios would also be well equipped with a non-symbolic commitment to trans inclusivity, including publicly available anti-oppression or equity policies that reflect those aims and promote wider advocacy.

---

24. See Lakshmi Nair, "When Even Spirit Has No Place to Call Home: Cultural Appropriation, Microaggressions, and Structural Racism in the Yoga Workplace." *Race and Yoga* 4, no. 1 (2019): 33-38, https://escholarship.org/uc/item/8mn5k1m1; Tobias Wiggins, "You Are Here: Exploring Yoga and the Impacts of Cultural Appropriation," YouTube video, 25:25, July 17, 2014, https://www.youtube.com/watch?v=3OoBaDt9cvQ.

Beyond preparing studios to be anti-oppressive, however, another necessary strategy to support folks with marginalized identities is to provide real, tangible space for their voices and experiences. If we are working within a setting that has persistently excluded transgender people, it will take time and effort to transform and rebuild trust. And a lot of this trust can only be established when those with privilege step aside while actively propping up the voices of those who have been silenced.

One way to go about this re-centering is through free or subsidized "queer and trans" yoga classes led by queer and trans identified people, like those I offer in Toronto, Ontario. These identity-based classes shift power hierarchies by putting marginalized people in paid[25] leadership positions, allowing them to co-envision a future, and facilitate their community's healing. When queer and trans people come together to breathe and move, the simplicity of being seen, recognized, and reflected can hold tremendous potential for self-expansion. In a social context where many of us still struggle to survive or thrive, it can be most powerful to be in a healing process collectively—no matter how that healing looks—be it falling apart, growing, disconnecting, reconciling, sweating it out, exploding in laughter, or opening a new gateway.

The systemic issues that transgender people face, whether in yoga studios or other social institutions, cannot be undone by wishing it to be so. It will take people who are willing to be accountable and humble, who are willing to move aside for others, to learn, and to facilitate a new vision for who belongs in a yoga community.

---

25. Another way that power dynamics appear is through the expectation that marginalized people provide these classes or educate those with privilege to be "better allies" through underpaid/unpaid labor.

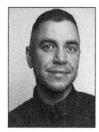

Tobias Wiggins, PhD is an assistant professor of women's and gender studies at Athabasca University, a social justice consultant, and a trauma-informed yoga instructor in Alberta, Canada. He's received several awards for his scholarship and activism, including Yoga Alliance Foundation's competitive Aspiring Yoga Teacher Scholarship, which is awarded to yoga practitioners with a high level of leadership with underserved populations. As a queer trans man, his community work aims to increase awareness of sociopolitical issues and actively challenge oppression. Visit tobywiggins.com for more.

# MY BUDDHA BODY

## *Michael Hayes*

As a large-bodied black man, I had to find my own way in yoga and my own way in the world.

My yoga practice began when I was going to massage school; I kept hearing about its benefits and finally decided to give it a try. I had actually tried yoga once before at Integral Yoga on Fourteenth Street: in those classes we would do a pose, then lie down, do a pose, then lie down, and so on. I thought it was interesting—relaxing—but it didn't really "stick" for me and I hadn't been back. But that's what I thought yoga was, so when I went to Jivamukti Yoga for the first time, the class basically kicked my ass.

I had never seen jump-backs before. I had never seen jump-throughs before. After the first sun salutation A and B, they all went into handstands in the middle of the floor, and I was pissed. I was a martial artist, I'd done dance and all sorts of stuff, and I said to myself, "I'm going to come back here afterward when I finish school because I refuse to let anything like this kick my ass."

I finished massage school, and I wanted to go back to Jivamukti, but I didn't have much money, so I decided I would try to do an exchange, like massage for yoga. I was told I could do karma yoga: if I cleaned up the studio, I could take classes in exchange for my work, but then the manager asked me how many times I'd taken classes. I told her only once, a year back, and she thought because I wasn't a regular, I couldn't be a karma yogi. At that very moment, she got locked out of her office and asked me if I could unlock her door. I asked her if she had a butter knife; she found one and I was able to open the door, and she agreed to let me do karma yoga!

I've been telling this story for close to twenty years now, and I never really realized until about five years ago how incredible that moment was: the door literally closes, I open it with a butter knife, and it opens me up to this system of yoga. That moment changed everything. I went to Jivamukti pretty much every morning, and that was my introduction to doing yoga. Now, I wasn't able to do all of the stuff other people were doing. Nobody but me was using blocks. And at a certain point I realized *I can't do any of this shit*. So I'd ask teachers, "How do I do these poses?" They said I should get more involved and to keep on trying, but that wasn't really working for me. I considered taking Jivamukti's teacher training because I wanted to understand what the teachers were thinking, but in the end, it was just way too expensive. I was only just beginning to build my massage practice.

But I wanted to explore yoga and I really wanted to explore working with props. The cofounder of Jivamukti, David Life, recommended the Sivananda teacher training in the Bahamas. I went and it was interesting, but with my background in massage and anatomy and my experience with Jivamukti, I had a certain way of thinking about movement, and I didn't understand the system there. I was happy with some of what I was getting intellectually, but I was very frustrated with what I was getting physically. What I really wanted to know is *why* people are doing certain things. Why do we have to do a sun salutation that way? What is the idea behind it? What is the purpose of a handstand? What is that doing for me? Ultimately, I felt discouraged because I wasn't getting the answers I needed.

For a year afterward I didn't go to any yoga classes, I just practiced on my own in the mornings, but at a certain point I got stuck; I couldn't go any further. Luckily, I knew a yoga teacher who needed massage therapy and we started doing exchanges. We worked together for about a year, and then I did her teacher training, which was an amazing experience because she brought different yogis in to talk about their process. It was exactly what I needed. After the training, I really wasn't thinking about becoming a teacher. I thought there was no way that anyone was going to hire a big black man to lead a yoga class and that my practice of yoga was very different from anything out there. I needed to go through different yoga practices, experiencing different modalities of yoga, to find my way into my own practice.

## How I Started Buddha Body Yoga

Eventually I studied with Leslie Kaminoff, who was working about three blocks away from me at the time. I did his Yoga for Anatomy course, and I learned why the breath is important and about the bandhas, the whole bit. And I took all of that and ran with it. I took what he gave me and I played with it, with my own body and with people I was working with. I started giving free private lessons because I wanted to understand what was going on in people's bodies. My curiosity soared.

At the time I was the only big person I ever saw in any classes. Iyengar, vinyasa, you name it. I would bring my own blocks and my own bolster. The teachers would look at me like I was absolutely crazy, but then they left me alone, which was good. I got to know the routines and the flows, and I eventually started teaching. More and more people came to me. And that's how I started my studio, Buddha Body Yoga. And then I was featured in an article in the *New York Times*, and the studio and my teaching began to gain recognition.

There were only a few people who were doing what I was doing then: teaching yoga for plus-sized people. And I wanted people to understand that I was committed to working with them *where they are* so they can develop their skills and have their own practice. It's a process and the end was, and still is, not as important to me as that beginning and middle. Process is of the utmost importance.

## The Power of Yoga

Yoga is powerful. I have done and still do therapy. I've done Al-Anon, Overeaters Anonymous, ACOA. I've done Gestalt. They all gave me tools to deal with certain things, but yoga opened me up in a brand-new way. I'll give you a story: At Jivamukti, I sometimes did two classes back-to-back. One day after I did two classes I walked out of the school, and I felt like something had left me. Something emotional, something really deep had left me. I don't know what it was, but I chilled out and let myself be who I was. I never forgot that. I've had little bits of that ever since.

It was an awakening, an awakening of the body sense rather than the mind sense. Because the body holds so much information, so much memory. With even a short amount of time to practice, you can recharge your way of thinking.

## Meditation and Ice Cream

What I've learned over the years is that yoga is not just about the poses. Meditation is the key. Take five or ten minutes, every three or four hours, every day. It's a great way to reorganize your intentions. It alters your belief systems of who you are and what you have and how to live. The resilience part of yoga is making time to do your practice. It's a conversation that happens *with your body*, and I'm not talking about in yoga and meditation *classes*. People have no problem going to class and letting somebody lead them; the challenge is for them to do their own practice. If you're not doing your own practice, if you're not playing with what's going on with your own body, you're watching television with your body as the television.

I went to a vipassana ten-day silent retreat when I was younger. The experience changed my life because of what happened in those ten days. All the stories that ran in my head from all the commercials I've ever seen on television, to all the stories of people in my life, the arguments—all of it came up, out, and through me. And the biggest thing was ... I wanted ice cream.

There I was in the meditation zone, and I'm seeing the ice cream in front of me and oh, it looks so good. Finally, I get out of there, I go to the ice cream place. I had ice cream in my hands, on the table, and I'm eating it and eating it … and it didn't taste as good as when it was in my mind. That was a game changer for me. It means there's a disconnect between what I think and feel and reality. I remembered how it tasted the first time, and I was going back trying to get that same taste.

## What I'd Love for My Community

I've seen so much change over the years in yoga, so much success. There are people out there now who are doing the plus-sized work. It's amazing, but what I'd really love is for us all to be together and talk about the physicality of yoga. There are some things that I'd love to rave about that we're doing and other things I'd love to challenge the community on to see if I can get them to change the way they're thinking about yoga, to move from the old paradigm to a new one.

I have questions for the community. Like are we engaging with our bellies in our yoga? Or are we using our arms and legs to avoid the belly? How are plus-sized people using the bandhas? That could be a whole conference. How do we get these areas to work *and* relax enough so the practice doesn't hurt our backs? The hips, the butt, and the belly work against us and support us at the same time. Imagine being able to play with your inversions to help you with your high blood pressure. Playing with rolling to rid the gas from your large intestines. To fart in your yoga class. That's what I want to talk about.

There's a quote by Octavia Butler that says, "All that you Change Changes you. The only lasting truth is Change. God is Change."[26] I believe that's true. That's one of the things that yoga has given me in a certain sense. In my struggle to develop my practice, I also have struggled to develop my own sense of what is mine.

Have I had trauma in my life? Yes. I'd say most people of color in America and most people of size have trauma in their lives. Does it define me? Yes. It does define me, but how I use it defines me more.

26. Octavia Butler, *Parable of the Sower* (New York: Warner Books, 1993), 2.

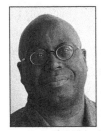

Michael Hayes, the proud owner of a "Buddha body," and Buddha Body Yoga in New York City, has more than twenty years' experience teaching and has studied extensively in the following traditions: Iyengar Yoga, Ashtanga Yoga, Thai Yoga, Om Vinyasa Yoga, and Yoga Anatomy. In addition, Michael has traveled regularly to Thailand to study with master teachers. His class will benefit anyone regardless of their individual anatomy, flexibility, age, or yoga background. Michael has also practiced massage for more than twenty years as a licensed massage therapist. Learn more at www.buddhabodyyoganyc.com.

# FROM VICIOUS CYCLES TO VIRTUOUS CYCLES: HEALING CHILDHOOD SEXUAL TRAUMA

## Susanna Barkataki

My partner would reach out to caress me, and I would startle, jump, and pull away.

As an adult survivor of childhood sexual assault, I became very disassociated from my body. From nightmares to headaches, social anxiety, and other disconnected behavior, it was clear that the past trauma I had experienced was impacting my life every single day.

Later, I learned this disassociation is a natural and healthy way to cope with traumatic situations in the moment; now many therapists call this the "submit" response. I'm glad I was able to disassociate during the trauma. But as I experienced later in life, as an adult in the present moment, the disassociation spread through many areas of my life. Even as I write this, I notice my attention wanting to drift away and disconnect.

I didn't know it at the time, but trauma affects the entire mind-body-spirit system.

As a young person, I walked around like I was a head with no body. I would walk around school lost in thought. I was covered in bruises from bumping into things—walls, tables, and chairs. I had lots of anxiety, a strong startle reflex that disrupted sleep, and dreams that I would wake from screaming.

In intimate relationships I was often replaying traumatic scenes or re-creating them. This led to unhealthy adult relationships as well.

It was only later that I learned that adult survivors of repeated childhood sexual trauma can experience post-traumatic stress disorder.

Like many of us, I was living life while I had many symptoms of PTSD. I was constantly on edge. My nervous system was ramped up. I was attending a great college and highly functioning, but I was a mess.

## Yoga Encounters, Release, and Integration

Though I had practiced yoga ethics and philosophy—yoga off the mat—with my family since I was young, when I finally got on a yoga mat in a college class, I lay in child's pose with tears coming down my face. Instead of feeling disconnected from my body, this was the first time I actually felt at home and connected within my own skin. I began to practice yoga asana more regularly, and each time I would find myself releasing through tears or breath.

I began a daily dhyana, or meditation and yoga practice, and the effects began to be noticeable.

I started observing that I wasn't bumping into things as much. I slept better and awoke screaming in the night much less. I began to feel my mind, body, and emotions integrating. I stopped putting myself in harm's way in unhealthy relationships because I was aspiring to practice ethical behavior and take care of myself well through practicing the yamas and niyamas, or inner and outer codes of yogic conduct. I began to take care of myself and speak lovingly toward myself and others. I began managing my energy, respecting others and myself in new ways.

A lot of this journey wasn't fully conscious. I was experiencing the healing through doing the practice. It was a journey of learning and discovery. I was healing internalized wounds as well, the parts that had felt that being Indian made me unworthy were healing as I used the practices from my roots and ancestors to heal me in the present moment.

Only later did I realize that I had come a long way from the traumatized and reactive person I had been. I began to have healthy relationships with myself, my friends, and even with a romantic partner.

The yoga was definitely working. So I had to ask myself, why does this work so well?

## My Experience of Yoga's Usefulness in Treating Trauma

Because yoga is a body-based practice, it helped me redefine and reconnect to a healthy relationship with the body I had been so disconnected from.

With the practice of moving and breathing in sync, my mind and body started to integrate as I learned to follow my own breath and be in the present moment.

Yoga helped me build a sense of connection to myself again. It helped me undo internalized oppression and unpack beliefs of my own or my culture's inferiority. Interestingly, this is the same practice Gandhi used in his Satyagraha movement to empower India to throw off British oppressive rule.

The practice worked inside and out. After some time, with practicing yoga and a focus on the breath, I was able to cultivate my ability to remain present with current experiences.

Yoga helped me realign my biorhythms. The tools of my practice gave me guidance to listen to the body and make choices that were more natural for me. Breathing and moving in slow postures like cat-cow allowed me to begin to create my own rhythms. This practice of creating rhythms, creating synchrony rather than dis-synchrony, finding one's own flow and rhythm in class, aided my everyday life.

Learning how to take my yoga off the mat with ayurveda allowed me to harmonize biorhythms such as eating, sleeping, and energy. The common dysregulation that can occur in these rhythms through trauma was healed and harmonized through practicing yogic lifestyle, asana, and pranayama or breathwork.

# From Vicious Cycles to Virtuous Cycles

My practice allowed me to have a transformative realization about how to turn this vicious cycle into a virtuous one.

It was the tenth day of a twelve-day silent meditation retreat, and the teacher was teaching us all about karma, impermanence, and letting go.

This teaching may not be for everyone. For me it was liberating.

As she was teaching about karma, she invited us to take 100 percent responsibility for the events in our lives. She said, even if not in this life, perhaps in another life you've done something that created the conditions even for the worst events that have happened to you. I could hear this, take responsibility, and actually not feel guilty or ashamed. It actually made me feel more powerful.

Perhaps there were actions that created the conditions for the abuse I experienced to occur. It became no longer about blame or shame. It was not my fault. It was not even the perpetrator's fault. He was clearly suffering and a survivor himself and barely an adult at that.

I understood that it was bigger than us and that the only way out of this cycle of harm was forgiveness and nonviolent action. Forgiveness allowed me to let go of the anger and resentment I was holding on to and actually allowed me to open into more peace within myself.

The teaching of ahimsa (nonviolence) and aparigraha (letting go of attachments), aided me in this transformation.

I became committed to transforming vicious cycles into virtuous ones through healing and transformation.

## Sharing the Journey of Healing

The practice of yoga and mindfulness has been a great journey of healing for me. But after getting enough stability in my own life, I realized that this work doesn't end with me. Using the tools that helped me to support others in their journey of recovery and healing became my calling.

A teacher by trade, I knew I wanted to share what was working so well for me. Through offering meditation groups and donation yoga, I began to teach what I had learned. It was at this moment that something became abundantly clear: The issues of abuse of power are systemic. I was not the only one healing trauma. Not by far. Many of my students had been in abusive relationships, had sexual trauma, or other traumas that they were healing from.

I started to see that it wasn't an accident. These are systemic problems and they need a systemic solution. Now, through trauma-informed yoga, I work with trauma survivors, we can turn vicious cycles into virtuous cycles. In my recent teacher training, cohorts and I work with students to teach the basics of asana, the philosophy of yoga, and the other eight limbs. We also include an analysis of colonization, power, privilege, and oppression as well as trauma-informed, healing-centered recovery and spiritual wellness and how we can use the powers we cultivate in our practice for the good of ourselves, others, and society. We tie yoga to social justice, healing ourselves as we work toward healing our world.

My hope is that more and more of us allow ourselves to face the traumas we may have experienced and heal them. We make room for helping others to heal when we heal ourselves. As more of us become aware of this system and change it, we even prevent the trauma from occurring in the first place.

I continue to heal myself as I share yoga, teaching others—particularly survivors of sexual trauma, partner abuse, or those with PTSD—how to breathe, release, reclaim, and live their power. Yoga and mindfulness have become, for me, some of the most effective ways of guiding people to reclaim internal power in order to move into healthy roles and relationships, have more fulfilling lives, and bring positive, transformative power into the world.

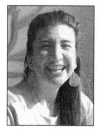

Susanna Barkataki is a teacher, inclusivity promoter, yoga culture advocate, and founder of Ignite Yoga & Wellness Institute, which has online and in-person trainings. Susanna has an honors degree from UC Berkeley and a master's in education, is an E-RYT 500-hour master teacher, a 500-hour certified ayurvedic practitioner, and a C-IAYT Yoga Therapist. Learn more at www.susannabarkataki.com and find out about online trainings at www.ignitebewell.com. Author photo by Samantha Santiago.

# YOGA TURNED MY BODY INTO A PLACE I COULD CALL HOME

## *Amber Karnes*

Hey y'all, my name is Amber, and I'm fat.

Yeah, fat. I'm plus-sized, big, chunky, curvy, plump, larger-bodied, fat. You can pick whatever word you prefer to describe my body. But I prefer the word fat.

Fat is a word that I've reclaimed as part of my identity. A word that for most of my life has been hurled at me as an insult: *fat*, the worst thing you can call a woman.

When I use the word fat, though, I don't want you to hear an insult. The word fat is a neutral descriptor to me. I'm fat. I am also a white woman, short, tattooed, green-haired (at the moment), a glasses-wearer, and thirty-six years old. When I say that I'm fat, I don't want you to hear any of the stigma, shame, or baggage that society attaches to that word. I'm just fat.

I wasn't a fat child, but I've been fat since my teenage years. I distinctly remember my weigh-in for the volleyball team at age fourteen: 212 pounds, and heavier than all but one girl on the team. (A valid reason for weighing high school volleyball players still escapes me.)

So, most of my life, I've been fat. And most of my life, I have hated my body. I saw my body as the enemy. It wouldn't obey. It wouldn't do what I desperately needed it to do (become thin). I saw my body as a project to constantly be improved, as something to be punished. Sometimes I saw my body as something to be ignored.

And at other times, my body was something I desperately wanted to be separate from. I wanted to believe that it had nothing to do with me (the real me, anyway).

## The Cultural Weight of Living in a Fat Body

Anyone who lives in a body that's the opposite of what society says is good, desirable, or worthy probably has felt that way. From the time I started to develop at an early age, it felt like my body was up for public comment and debate from leering boys and men who yelled at me on the street. When I put on weight as a teenager and firmly landed in the category of *fat girl*, the type of attention shifted.

Street harassment changed from catcalls, whistles, car horns, and "Hey, baby!" into moo-ing, "Whale!" or "Fat bitch!" and trash or drinks thrown at me from car windows. Nowadays, I experience most of my harassment online. Having the audacity to be a fat person who publicly exists without apologizing for her body means I spend time deleting violent, bullying, fatphobic comments from my social media accounts and inbox on a daily basis.

When folks who don't fit the dominant beauty ideal are represented in media, we are rarely shown in a positive light. Growing up, when I saw a fat woman on TV, in the movies, or portrayed in books, she was never the successful protagonist. She was the butt of a joke, sloppy, lazy, chasing a man who didn't want her, clueless, stupid. If a fat character did get portrayed positively, it was through a redemptive "before and after" weight loss narrative. The message was clear (from society and from media): If you get thin, you get the guy, the cool clothes, the popular friends, the awesome career. If you stay fat, you get shame, ridicule, and will probably die alone.

Author Junot Diaz said, "If you want to make a human being into a monster, deny them, at the cultural level, any reflection of themselves."[27] And denying marginalized folks any positive reflection of themselves is one way that the culture withholds power. Society's messages about beauty and worth get reinforced. And systems of oppression (capitalism, patriarchy, white supremacy) function best when we internalize that oppression, that feeling of inferiority.

When we internalize oppression, when we police *ourselves* by treating our bodies as problems to be solved and projects to be worked on, when we make self-loathing into a full-time job, no man on the street has to yell, "UGLY!" from a car window. *We know.* Deep down, we already know, and we understand that we are expected to have an apology for our very existence always at the ready.

There's plenty of peer-reviewed, empirical evidence about the treatment that fat folks receive in our culture. Fat folks face a staggering amount of weight bias in the medical industry,[28] which literally is a life or death situation since our pain, symptoms, and requests for treatment are routinely denied or ignored, which can lead to misdiagnosis and death. Fat women are less likely to be hired[29] than their thin counterparts, and if they are hired, are also paid less.[30] If you happen to end up in court as a fat person, there's a good chance you won't get a fair trial.[31]

27. Brian Donohue, "Pulitzer Prize-Winning Author Junot Diaz Tells Students His Story," NJ.com, last modified January 19, 2019, https://www.nj.com/ledge rlive/2009/10/junot_diazs_new_jersey.html.

28. Kelly Coffey, "Weight Bias in Health Care: The Shocking Ways Large Women Are Mistreated by Health-Care Providers," SELF, Conde Nast, July 18, 2017, https://www.self.com/story/weight-bias-and-health-care.

29. Stuart W. Flint, Martin Šadek, Sonia C. Codreanu, Vanja Ivić, Colene Zomer, and Amalia Gomoiu, "Obesity Discrimination in the Recruitment Process: 'You're Not Hired!'," *Frontiers in Psychology* 7, no. 647 (May 2016): n.p., https://doi.org/10.3389/fpsyg.2016.00647.

30. Charles L. Baum II and William F. Ford, "The Wage Effects of Obesity: A Longitudinal Study," Health Economics 13, no. 9 (September 2004): 885-899, https://doi.org/10.1002/hec.881.

31. Natasha A. Schvey, Rebecca M. Puhl, K. A. Levandoski, and K. D. Brownell, "The Influence of a Defendant's Body Weight on Perceptions of Guilt," *International Journal of Obesity* 37, no. 9 (September 2013):1275-1281, https://doi.org/10.1038/ijo.2012.211.

And when body size intersects with race or gender, the rate of discrimination increases.[32]

It takes a toll, being fat in a world where fat bodies are pathologized on first glance, where there is a "war on obesity," where fat bodies are up for public comment and debate. The fact that society believes a fat body is a signal of moral failure means that fat people endure bullying, stigma, and shame on a daily basis, both on an individual and a systemic, societal basis.

## "Amber, I'd Like to Introduce You to Your Body." — Yoga

So, it was with this experience and awareness of my fat body that I walked into my first yoga class in my early twenties. I was on some big weight loss project at the time, and I'd heard that yoga was something I should do at the gym on my rest days—that it didn't really "count" as exercise, but I would still burn calories. So off to yoga I went, to obediently burn more calories. I don't remember anything much about that first class, besides being the only fat person in the room. What I do remember was leaving the class, walking to my car, driving away, getting on the interstate to go home, and about ten minutes into my drive, the familiar mental soundtrack starting back up.

Maybe you've experienced this soundtrack too, that voice in the back of your mind that second-guesses everything you do, tells you you aren't good enough, reminds you of that stupid thing you said or did, and constantly judges and casts shame onto your body.

What I realized was that if the ol' judgment reel had started back up, that meant it had stopped. Even for a few minutes, my mind had quieted itself and I had spent those minutes not thinking about or judging my body or myself. This was new! I was eager to repeat this experiment, so I went back to class. A few classes more, and I was hooked.

32. Jennifer A. Ailshire, and James S. House, "The Unequal Burden of Weight Gain: An Intersectional Approach to Understanding Social Disparities in BMI Trajectories from 1986 to 2001/2002," *Social Forces* 90 (2): 397–423, https://doi.org/10.1093/sf/sor001.

In yoga, I was really *in* my body for the first time in a long time. I was experiencing joyful movement, which I hadn't felt since I was a child. Thanks to the trainer and his terribly inaccurate description of what to expect from yoga, I hadn't approached it the same way I approached most exercise. I allowed myself to have an embodied experience. I wasn't punishing, ignoring, or hating my body during yoga class. And I left class feeling calmer, less anxious, and more comfortable in my skin.

When I began practicing yoga, the teachers didn't know what the heck to do with me. Even though my body wasn't making many of the shapes that they were asking of it, in most of the classes I went to, I was ignored. There were no modifications offered. Sometimes they'd say, "Use a block if you need one," with no instruction on what to do with the block. Surely the teachers could see that I couldn't do some of what they were asking, and yet, they ignored me.

Looking back now, being ignored for a few years of my practice was a gift, because it meant that I had to be creative and have agency when it came to my practice. Back then, there were no online videos explaining how to modify poses. There were no blogs or podcasts about diversity in yoga. There were no yogis who looked like me with hundreds of thousands of followers on Instagram. And in class, no one was telling me why I couldn't step my foot forward between my hands to get from down dog into a lunge or how to get there in a different way, so I had to figure it out myself.

I won't say that my practice was always pretty, but I will say that it was *mine*.

I was confronted with the reality of my body during these classes, as my belly, thighs, breasts, and butt got in my way in poses, and I had to be creative about how to approximate the shapes that the other students were making. I started moving my stuff out of the way.

I discovered one day that if I put my hands on my body and physically moved my belly out of the way of my thigh, I could sink deeper into a lunge. I figured out that if I shoved my breast underneath my arm I could reach across my body in a seated twist. I realized that if I tucked my belly up and back toward my pelvis in a forward fold, not only could

I move deeper into the pose, I instinctively understood what the teacher meant by "hinge at the hips." I learned to walk my hands back to my feet in down dog instead of stepping forward into a lunge.

I got to know my body. I became more physically fluent and present in my body. And that changed everything.

## Yoga Turned My Body into a Place I Could Call Home

Mindful movement made me more physically certain of myself. Yes, my body got stronger. Yes, I learned to make the shapes that the teacher was asking for, and I learned to move with intention. But my mind got stronger as well.

My yoga practice made me sure—made me know in my bones—that my body was a powerful, good, and safe place to be. That embodied knowledge was reinforced by the things I was learning outside of class.

My discovery of yoga and mindfulness happened at the same time I discovered the fat acceptance movement and the concept of body positivity. I started learning more about systems of oppression and the construct of beauty currency. I learned that the diet industry is a $60 billion per year industry with a product that has a 95 percent failure rate.[33] I discovered the Health at Every Size® approach to wellness, which is based in the scientific evidence that our best chance at health is through cultivating healthy habits, regardless of body size.

I quit dieting. I gave up intentional weight loss as a pursuit. I discovered that my thoughts about body size had not come from a place of truth inside me but from society's expectations and narrowly defined beauty standards.

As I developed a new relationship with my body, the locus of control moved from an extrinsic place to an intrinsic place.

Food was no longer about some prescribed calorie count, approved list of foods, or cutting out food groups (extrinsic); it was about listening to my body's signals of hunger, fullness, satiety, and pleasure (intrinsic).

33. Esther Rothblum, "Slim Chance for Permanent Weight Loss," *Archives of Scientific Psychology* 6 no. 1 (2018): 63-69, http://dx.doi.org/10.1037/arc0000043.

Movement was no longer punitive, something I had to do to "earn" my food or something I did to change my body (extrinsic); instead it was about improved mental and physical health (intrinsic), feeling joyful in my body, feeling strong, and feeling good.

When I looked in the mirror I no longer picked apart my appearance to find every flaw or what was lacking according to society's beauty standards (extrinsic); instead I was able to appreciate my body for what it could do, how it could be my ally, my partner in crime, in the awesome process of being Amber (intrinsic).

As I changed my thoughts about my body, food, health, movement, and self-worth, I stopped hating my body. I learned to claim the space I took up in the world without shame. I was able to fully embody my power, make bold moves, and live life out loud.

## Body Positive Yoga: Honoring the Body You Bring to the Mat Today

I decided to take yoga teacher training about seven years into my practice—not to become a teacher but to deepen my personal practice and learn "the rest of yoga" outside just the poses. But during teacher training it occurred to me that if I'd had the experience in yoga classes of being ignored and left to fend for myself for years, then other people were having that experience too.

Many of my students who had a bad first experience in yoga never went back until they found me (or another teacher who looks like them and understands their bodies). When they were ignored in class, they didn't assume the teacher didn't know how to work with them. They just saw a class full of people doing what the teacher asked while they got no acknowledgment that they were having a different experience. They felt uncomfortable, maybe they injured themselves, but in any case, they definitely left the class "knowing for a fact" that their body was wrong for yoga. Everyone else could do the poses as the teacher demonstrated them, but they couldn't, so their body was wrong.

My teaching is about helping my students understand that their bodies aren't wrong for yoga, that their bodies aren't problems to be solved. It's about sharing the life-changing benefits of embodiment that have been so powerful for me. It's about helping them have a positive experience of the body they have today through movement and mindfulness (with a healthy dose of context and awareness of the systems of oppression that get us messed up about bodies in the first place).

My work these days is also in training other yoga teachers how to work with folks who are traditionally underserved in the yoga world: folks in larger bodies, older folks, disabled folks, folks with mobility limitations, and raw beginners.

I truly believe that right now, the best way I can be of service in life is by helping folks to make peace with their bodies.

I believe that if we reclaim our time, money, and mental energy from diet culture and a constant obsession on our "flaws," then we can realize our power, potential, and fire. We can and will change the world. When we can exist in our bodies without shame or apology, we will each realize the unique gifts that only we can offer to the world.

## "She Really Let Herself Go."

There's this phrase that's invoked when women gain weight, quit wearing makeup, stop dyeing their hair, or basically stop trying to assimilate to the dominant culture's beauty standards.

*"Wow, she really let herself go."*

I used to cringe at that phrase. But nowadays, I will totally cop to that (letting myself go).

You're damn right I let myself go.

I let myself go from upholding systems of oppression that get to deny or grant us worth based on beauty or productivity instead of our humanity.

I let myself go from the constant shame and hate, the internalized inferiority of my body, of the feeling of wanting to escape my own skin and bones.

I let myself go from buying into a system that profits off my dissatisfaction with my body.

I let myself go from chronic dieting, gaining and losing weight over and over again, obsessing over every bite of food or calorie burned.

I let myself go from attitudes and paradigms that turned food into an anxiety-producing experience or a moral failing instead of something to be enjoyed.

I let myself go from experiencing movement and exercise as a punitive act fraught with disappointment and missed expectations. I let myself go from never being able to enjoy moving my body.

I let myself go from the constant mean girl in my head who yells all day long that I'm not good enough.

I let myself go from postponing "living my real life" until a day when I "finally lost the weight."

I did let myself go. I got free.

(Let's get free, y'all.)

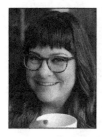

Amber Karnes is the founder of Body Positive Yoga. She's a ruckus maker, yoga teacher, social justice advocate, and a lifelong student of her body. She's the co-creator of Yoga for All teacher training, an Accessible Yoga trainer and board member, and a sought-after expert on the topics of accessibility, authentic marketing, culture shifting, and community building. She lives in Baltimore, Maryland, with her husband, Jimmy. You can find her at bodypositiveyoga.com.

Author photo by Hidden Exposure Photography.

# SOMEWHERE UNDER THE RAINBOW

## *Rachel Otis*

Among childhood memories of building blanket forts and pretending to skip down the yellow brick road hid the shadows that came alive at night and danced on my wall and inside my body—vivid memories of the times I would stand in front of the tall bathroom mirror as a little girl, and eventually a young woman, pushing, pulling, and pinching my belly rolls together. I imagined what it would look like to have a flat stomach, wishing passionately that I could just chop those parts off— the parts of myself that caused shame, that made me feel "other than" in a world of sameness.

The process of becoming the adult that I am today has been complicated and arduous; it has also been full of wonder, support, authenticity, healing, love, and opportunities to create positive change in the world. It's been a journey of learning to embrace myself as I am by embodying self-love, which has involved carving out a distinctive life path all my own.

### Early Years: Integrating and Disintegrating

During childhood and into adolescence, I was constantly fluctuating between wanting to fit in and desiring to exude my uniqueness. Over the years, it would become increasingly clear that no one single group of humans could necessarily resonate with every part of my being. I am composed of an array of identities; the term for this I now know is intersectionality: Native American, English, French, Sicilian, Russian, German, Jewish, and Christian. My upbringing was mixed religiously, spiritually, and I attended Catholic school in New Hampshire to top it off! In my adulthood I also now proudly identify as Queer. I am not one thing, I am many.

The resulting feeling is a confusing mix of oppositions: my body has been, and I suspect always will be, simultaneously hyper visible and invisible. Nothing that speaks to my soul can be seen on my person by the eyes of others. What can be seen, however, is my bigger body size, which has led to a variety of reactions from others over the years— almost every single one of them projections of societal fears, desires, or both, none of which speak to my value as a human being. Although I had incredible family support, the majority of messaging I received from the world at large was that my body wasn't my own.

In fact, I have made the point many times that most womyns'[34] bodies bear the brunt of expectations related to societal norms and capitalistic, patriarchal depictions associated with beauty and self-worth, which can be inherently traumatizing to our mind-bodies. Seemingly from birth (and arguably even long before), the door is left wide open for others' opinions on our bodies: what they should be and what they shouldn't.

It feels important to note here that all of the above is wisdom I've accumulated in my adult years after somatic, therapeutic self-work—my younger self knew nothing of the truths I now hold dear.

When I was young and highly sensitive, I internalized the very essence of others' projections until I believed them to be my own (like many children before and after me). Unfortunately, I swallowed them whole, soaking them into my gut, my very core. The taste of these pro-

---

34. I personally choose to not use "man" or "men" as the base or root word in my languaging in the same way I don't use a presumed "he" as the default pronoun in my writing. For me, restructuring words in this way speaks to the way I work as an intersectional feminist and activist.

jections was so palpable that it takes all of my strength to even speak my truth on them now; sometimes I still feel their bitterness lingering in my mouth.

## Externalizing Fat Phobia

From receiving subtle or strong media messaging surrounding body image ideals, experiencing cruelty from schoolyard bullies, dreading group weigh-ins at the nurse's office, and overhearing other womyn body shame themselves, the constant message I was receiving was that something was wrong with me. However, the still-fitting truth of the matter is that something was and still is very wrong with society. That thing is fat phobia, or the pervasive, socially created, and often internalized fear of fat. Of course, this falls among other things—including pervasive racism, heterosexism, xenophobia, misogyny, and ableism just to name a few.

## Societal Creation and Perpetuation of "One Size Fits All" Mentalities

If you are someone who moves through the world with an able body, thin privilege, or both, you may not have noticed many oppressive structural barriers put in place against disabled bodies, fat bodies, or both, although they know this daily lived reality all too well. Take for example the messaging that a classroom full of size-restrictive desks and chairs sends to a child who feels cramped sitting in their desk every single day: you're other than, your body doesn't belong here, you take up too much space. A child is much less likely than an adult to be able to question this messaging or the societal structures that created it. One reason of course being that children aren't necessarily taught that they can question society. This subsequently creates the illusion that every human should fit into this "one size fits all" structure, which of course is a myth again rooted in capitalism and patriarchy. Now, expand this example to sports and school uniforms, dance and Halloween costumes, bus seats, clothing sizes, media representation and consumption, and those dreaded national fitness tests.

## Waging War Within

As childhood quickly morphed into adolescence, the relationship I had with my body continued to become more distanced and disconnected. So much so that I even started to feel my body was an entity separate from and against me rather than one that literally supported my every move. Transitioning to high school, I found myself more easily aligning with society's projections about my body, which further reinforced the feeling that my body was the enemy. I often felt angry at my body, as well as hurt and betrayed by it. And by the end of my freshman year, I experienced an extremely painful shift in my lived bodily experience.

After months of hiding symptoms that I found too shameful and embarrassing to tell anyone about, due to the fact that they're bathroom-related (and again not socially acceptable to discuss), I could no longer function and began a series of invasive medical tests, which culminated in a diagnosis of Crohn's disease. I will never forget sitting anxiously in the doctor's office waiting for her to reveal what the tiny camera squeezed inside my intestines had discovered. In her harsh words, as she actually showed me pictures of the inside of my own gut, "You have the angriest looking colon I've ever seen!" The words didn't land as metaphorically with me then as they do now, but upon years of self-reflection and a lived and learned deep knowledge and understanding of how Crohn's disease manifests in my body, I am now extremely fascinated with the fact that the exact part of my body that I did experience deep anger with, the part that I wanted to cut off, to disappear, in fact and biological reality, began attacking itself. As an autoimmune illness, that is exactly what Crohn's disease does: it represents my body attacking itself—specifically my colon, intestines, and gut.

Had I internalized and channeled so much hatred inwardly to that part of my body that it ultimately resulted in this often-debilitating disease? The truth is I will never fully know the answer to that question, especially as much Crohn's research is still left to be done and much is tied to genetics and environment. However, I will never rule that out as a personal life lesson meant to be further explored and healed.

What I do know for sure about Crohn's disease is the following: it is chronic and represents ongoing lived trauma to my body. I have now lived half of my life not simply battling it but coexisting with and learning from it. Its symptoms are often deemed embarrassing or unacceptable to talk about in our society (including vomiting, diarrhea, intense stomach pain, nausea, fatigue, internal blood loss, and joint aching), it is often invisible to others, and it is extremely difficult to explain or understand fully, as it can manifest in various ways in different bodies. I have been receiving infusions of medication every two months via IV for the whole of my experience with the disease, which often relieves my Crohn's symptoms but unfortunately can cause some additionally unpleasant ones, as it serves to actually suppress my overactive immune system (leaving me vulnerable to germs, sickness, and infection).

I have also experimented with and utilized alternative forms of healing, including a gluten-free and whole-foods-based way of eating, which when adhered to truly improved my daily functioning and overall quality of life. I do approach this much differently than a diet, however, as I view them to be just another form of body terrorism against fat people in our society (which I have personally survived too much of in my lifetime).

By learning to manage my symptoms, I was beginning a new conversation with my body, one focused on healing that required me to slow down and actually listen to all parts of my mind-body. This would continue to grow and flourish after I found my yoga practice.

## Rooting in Tree Pose

Flashing past my undergraduate experience, which included a major in psychology, minor in English, and concentration in art history and quantum theory (not to mention the expansion of my own personal consciousness through an array of diverse friendships) brings us to a more current-day perspective on my life. Post graduating, I wasn't certain how I wanted to focus my studies into my career, but I was absolutely certain that I wanted to branch out from my New England roots to live precisely three-thousand miles away in the place that I had fallen in love with: Venice Beach, California.

By way of universal connection while visiting LA, I was introduced to Hala Khouri, who became not only my employer, but my mentor, and truly like family. She sparked a deeper sense of inspiration already resonating within me, being the first trauma-informed yogi and somatic therapist I had ever met. Although the media perpetuates images of yoga that are homogenous and ultimately harmful (almost exclusively depicting highly flexible, exceptionally strong, and "fit" practitioners who neatly conform to societal beauty standards), Hala came to represent yoga in a form that felt digestible and actually supportive for me.

Students were invited into the room exactly as we were, free of expectation, and the teacher held no expectations or judgments—allowing us to witness her authenticity while modeling the co-creation of space with her students, and creatively using inclusive languaging. As I became more familiar with her trauma-informed practice of holding space for others, I began to unlock deeper understandings of how to hold space for myself. I began honoring my body's strengths and accepting the many painful areas I still had to make peace with.

## Embodying Warriors I, II, and III!

While I was beginning to tap into my own body's abilities and learning to resource through breath, I was simultaneously and separately being introduced to the world of fat positivity and activism. This was a world I had previously known nothing of. A world that consists of the liberation and celebration of fat bodies, reclaiming the term "fat" in an empowered way, as it has been ingrained as negative in us for so long.

This was happening during a time when my internalized fat phobia was still so deep and unrecognizable that I even feared claiming the term feminist (due to the stereotypes associated in particular with being a feminist and having a fat body, but also because I was surrounded by whitewashed feminism as opposed to the real intersectional feminism I now know and celebrate) and still wouldn't have dreamed that my self of today could wear a crop top with skintight leggings proudly to the grocery store, let alone manage a supported handstand. I was, however, learning to find peace inside what could have been previously described as the battle zone of my body; a truce was soon on the horizon.

Enter: yoga, allowing me to establish a new (loving and forgiving) relationship with myself and a body that I previously thought only knew how to attack itself. Slowly, my practice became about the in-between spaces, more embodied contemplative moments. Could I dare to let myself feel free enough to try a new, challenging balance pose with the potential to fall? And if I did fall could I be ok with that? Could I learn the boundaries around my own pain and let myself surrender when I needed to? Was I able to let go of worrying about what anyone other than myself was doing? It was a gradual process of learning how to make peace with all that I was and all that I am. Combining this with engaging in somatic therapy led me to the current branch of my life's path: a somatic therapist leading a private practice, helping individuals and groups in-person, online, and worldwide.

Somatic therapy can be described as a wholistic and alternative therapeutic approach in which the mind-body connection is explored through various modalities such as supportive touch, mindfulness, guided meditation, exploring repeated gestures and held postures, movement expressions, vocalizations, visualizations, sensory awareness, yoga, music, and art (among many other things), connecting the client with their resources, cultivating coping tools, and co-creating new pathways for their behaviors to manifest.

## Making the Invisible Visible

My work as a somatic therapist has become serendipitously intertwined with the work I have engaged in as a body advocate, writer, and creative director, where I have been entrenched in social justice activism through the sharing of radical truths. To reach a wider audience, I also spearheaded and created specialized self-love campaigns, such as #BeyondBeauty and #FuckFatPhobia. I am also now a proud member of the Yoga and Body Image Coalition, the Off the Mat, Into the World community, am a certified yoga teacher myself, and along with my partner have created "SOGA" (a somatics and yoga slow flow model). Thanks to the connection of radical yogis, I have been exposed to specialized classes for bigger-bodied humans taught by wonderful bigger-bodied teachers. Many of these teachers have become colleagues with whom

I then had the honor of co-facilitating workshops. Being surrounded by somatically resonate bodies and likewise supporting them in their practice has helped me resonate with my own even deeper.

Not only was this surrounding of bodies occurring inside the yoga studio, but almost magically, larger-bodied yogis began representing themselves and being represented more on social media. Having a daily visual source of support to anchor to is also a unique and precious gift to be given—suddenly I began witnessing bodies similar to mine moving in ways I had been taught to believe were impossible—from full-on headstands to deep backbends and the gentle poses in between; I was in awe and joy.

It was through yoga that I learned that the healing power of safer spaces is not to be treated lightly. After years of various holding patterns denoting my desire to take up as little space as possible, I found liberation through claiming what I'd always wanted and needed: self-love and self-acceptance.

I have since come to have an acceptance-turned-love affair with the thickness of my own thighs and the softness of every roll, cellulite dimple, and stretch mark! I have dared to frolic freely on beaches from east to west coasts in nothing but a bikini. I have mastered the art of siding with my body against the negativity of others while allowing it to soak-in the positivity of others as well. I now know that my body really is an integral part of my wholistic self, my home during my brief time here on earth. I will continue to weave my new-found love of self into the very fabric of our collective consciousnesses by solidifying it in these written words as my lived truth. Thank you to all who receive them as such; they are my gift to you.

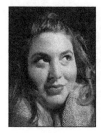

Rachel Otis is a somatic therapist, activist, and writer who works directly with the mind-body connection, infusing sessions, retreats, and articles with radical self-love, exploration, and expression, and providing healing pathways of somatically oriented coping tools and resources (including yoga, art, supportive self-touch, joyful movement, guided meditation, and breathing techniques). She is passionate about creating a more sustainable, socially just future by infiltrating oppressive systems to create change from the inside out for ALL bodies! Sliding scale and tele-therapy sessions available worldwide. You can reach out to her at www .rachelotistherapy.blog and connect with her on Instagram at @somewhere_under_the_rainbow.

Author photo by Katelyn Scott Photography.

# MY OWN HERO: HEALING MY INNER BLACK GAY CHILD

*Dorian Christian Baucum*

"Take those motherfucking boots off, boy! You want to grow up to be a faggot?" a tall, thick-bodied, husky-voiced, ashy caramel-colored seventeen-year-old yelled as a warning for the entire neighborhood to hear. His face was shaped like a lion's face and was pained with anger. His buddies were laughing like a bunch of hyenas, shaking their heads wide-eyed at me in disbelief. But he was dead serious.

A basketball on his hip, Alonzo and his friends had finally caught my four-year-old frame alone, switching and shaking my hips around in a pair of brown leather women's knee-high, zip-up, high-heeled go-go boots on my family's front porch on their way to hang out at his house after a ball game.

A working-class neighborhood of a predominately black Northwest Washington, DC, where people had raised their children and then watched their children raise children, everybody knew everybody else. Everybody knew the neighborhood kids and everything about them. For instance, people knew that I was being raised in a house full of women and lived next door to a house full of women as well—

a divorced woman and her five daughters who'd become extended family to us.

I'd often go into these women's closets that smelled of a flowery blend of their perfumes and leather from all the amazing shoes and boots they owned and pick out a pair to wear. It was one of my favorite pastimes.

Only around four or five years old, I would simply play in them by myself on the front porch. They'd ride all the way up to my waist. When the teen startled me, I was in my own world, perhaps emulating one of the women I lived with or had seen in the neighborhood or on TV and the way they walked. I don't remember everything about that moment clearly, but I do remember it was a summer evening. The sun was going down on our neighborhood. Our neighbors were probably sitting on the porches of houses they owned or watering their lawns. The doors to row houses were wide open like they always were with sounds from televisions and the smell of dinner being prepared coming through screen doors to my highly sensitive ears and nose.

Had the women who cared for me been in earshot at that moment, Alonzo would have never had the guts to say to me what he said, let alone yell at me like he did. Perhaps my female protectors were inside laughing too loudly, getting their hair pressed and curled for dates. Perhaps Alonzo had always wanted to say something to me about me playing in women's boots and finally had a clear opportunity to take his shot on this particular day.

I remember him, a giant compared to me, yelling like he was going to kick my ass. His voice was loud. And his voice let me—and everybody in the neighborhood—know that he was not going to stand for that kind of behavior from a male on his block because what I was doing was not what little boys should do. And I guess he felt it was his job to let me know.

I know people heard him, but nobody interfered to refute what he said or defend me from his verbal assault. More than likely because he was only voicing a concern that everybody had about me.

After a tense moment, Alonzo released an angry hiss from his mouth then he and his crew walked away.

I remember the shame and embarrassment I felt in my little four-year-old body. From that day forward, I would always feel a sense of disdain from males, young and old, in my neighborhood for my "softness" and my inability to live up to what everybody's idea of what an All-American black boy should be. Up until that point, I don't remember anyone raising his or her voice at me like that. I didn't know anything about what boys should be doing and what girls should be doing at that age; I didn't know anything about being gay or effeminate at that age. All I knew was that I was doing what made my heart happy. None of the women who loved me had told me it was wrong. To them, it was probably harmless for a little boy to play like that. But Alonzo and his buddies knew that this behavior was an indicator of something more malignant in the world of boys and men.

Throughout my childhood, I'd betray males in my neighborhood time and time again with this kind of "sissy-like," "soft" behavior.

I'd betray them just by being myself.

My entire childhood and teenage years would be filled with male figures in my life letting me know—either with a look or verbally—that there was something very wrong with me.

## The All-American Black Boy

Where I grew up, men were expected to act like men and little boys were expected to act like little boys. During the '80s and '90s, statistically, most young black men would be involved in some kind of street violence and would also spend some part of their lives incarcerated. So many black fathers, grandfathers, and uncles who had connections to young boys had to have it in their minds to groom young men that could not only survive the violent streets of Washington, DC, but that could also survive jail.

I was also a light-skinned kid. So there was even more reason for concern because light-skinned, high-yellow boys were seen as weaker. And the men I knew weren't having any soft-acting, high-yellow, black boys coming out of my neighborhood if they could help it. They had to make sure that I would be strong. "You got to be all boy! You got to be the All-American black boy!" was what a substitute gym teacher in my elementary school would say to us male youth often, his eyes focused mostly on me, it seemed.

As we lined up and filed out of the school gym, a classmate's grandfather that volunteered with the physical education program whispered to me as I walked by him, "Every soldier, every hero, finds his own glory, young man. You'll find your own glory!"

He seemed to be speaking directly to my wounded heart. I guess he saw the insecurity on my face. It's like he was telling me that despite what the substitute gym teacher had just said, that it was all right to be different from the other boys. Like many elder black men in our community, he'd proudly served as a lieutenant in World War II. Having led so many different kinds of men with so many different temperaments into battle, perhaps he had firsthand knowledge that surviving a war depended upon much more than physical prowess. I felt like this elder was letting me know that he saw my uncertainty and that I was going to be okay. Even though I didn't fit the image being projected onto all of us, better days were coming for kids like me.

The All-American black boy rode mopeds and dirt bikes. The All-American black boy could handle himself with his fists if someone disrespected him. The All-American black boy played sports, knew his way up and down a basketball court, and knew how to catch a football. The All-American black boy was a champion. The All-American black boy was a source of pride for the men in his community.

I never really took a liking to any of those things.

By my last year in elementary school, I knew that I was gay. I also knew that I couldn't tell anyone.

I played with the girls. I jumped double-dutch. I read books.

I was jumping rope with a group of girls in an alley behind my house one summer day when the words "That boy ain't gonna shit! He's gonna be gay," directed at me from the mouth of a loud intoxicated man out of a car window, hit me like a brick.

Even though there were always slivers of inspiration that would bolster my hope for better days in the future, like the grandfather in my gym class whispering to me, for the most part, the words coming from the mouths of men I looked up to devastated my young spirit and my confidence. I would go through my days and nights with those words echoing through my head. I'd look at other boys my age and wish I could be more like them and less like me.

Many young boys' reactions to the pressure to be manlier would have been to become overly masculine to win the approval of others they looked up to. But that wasn't my nature.

I was a gentle spirit. I had a poetic soul.

By the time I reached my teen years, I felt rejected and alone.

There were no LGBTQ clubs at DC area high schools. There were no gay pride parades happening in Washington, DC that I knew of. There were no same-sex couples raising children that were visible. They were not preaching inclusivity in the church that I went to.

If you were a gay kid growing up in Washington, DC in the '80s and early '90s, you were on your own.

There were many days when I just didn't want to live anymore.

Once I hit puberty, I began to pull away from friendships with males and females.

I didn't go out partying like other teens did. I just focused on academics.

I'd check out a book each week from the library to read during the long bus rides out of my neighborhood to attend magnet schools that I'd been accepted to in downtown Washington, DC. I'd become what people may consider a "gifted child," and that got me into schools away from my neighborhood. Away from anyone who really knew me, I spent time on the bus with my head buried in books communing with some of the most inspirational minds to ever live. And that's exactly what a young gay kid like me needed: inspiration.

James Baldwin, Maya Angelou, Richard Wright, Langston Hughes, the voice of Malcolm X through Alex Haley's book, Alice Walker— these folks became my allies. These were black writers who wrote mostly about their experiences with racial discrimination in America. But they also wrote very candidly about their experiences as children coming of age and how painful experiences shaped them into activists and advocates for the underdogs of this world. I could relate to them.

They weren't talking about being gay, but they were talking about being black and being different and oppressed. They were talking about how black people deserved better, how difference deserved to be celebrated, how difference deserved a voice. Since they were poets and writers, they did not all fit the stereotypes of what men should be (or women should be, for that matter), but they were successful and powerful.

Their books taught me that I could pour everything that I was going through as a teen into the arts. I could convert my pain into creativity, into creative projects. And that's exactly what I did.

I joined drama clubs, signed up for speech competitions, went away for summers to study in academic programs, and I began to shine in those areas. So much so that I began to win the approval of many people in my community.

As a teen, my love for the arts and books took me all over the country and eventually away from the streets of my hometown to college. It was in Boston while in college that I was able to find the space to allow my true identity to begin to come out.

But, coming out of the closet was just the first step. It would take nearly two decades for me to get to a place where I could deal with the pain of the childhood rejection I experienced. Yoga would be a conduit for that healing.

"You are enough." That's what yoga says. "Your life matters. You are special. You are a hero on your own journey. Come as you are. Accept yourself for who you are!"

No one had ever said that to me quite the way yoga teachers had.

Or maybe I was just at a point in my life—around forty years old—where I was ready to step more fully into myself. Even though I had achieved so much and come so far as an adult—I'd become a pharmacist, an actor, and a singer-songwriter living in Los Angeles, CA—my past, full of childhood rejection, had been trying to catch up with me. The traumatized child in me had been screaming for my attention through my adult years. Yoga—a tool that I did not have as a gay child growing up on the streets of Washington, DC—I now had. I was in a position in my life to utilize and take full advantage of it.

When I first started doing yoga, I used it as a way to relax for my artistic work. But I was also using it to try to stand out. I was trying to do it "right," trying to be a "good student." This was a survival mechanism that had gained me a certain amount of success in life, but it was also a symptom of something deeper: I was running away from a sense of inferiority. Men create hierarchies and gay men exist very low on those hierarchies. Once I realized that I had been subconsciously carrying around a false sense of inferiority for more than three decades, I really began to open up to allow my true self onto the mat and into my life. And that's when the practice of yoga really began to be a source of healing for me.

Yoga brings me to a place where I can watch my thoughts and separate out the voices in my head. I can distinguish between the abusive voices—the ones put there by society and some of the men I grew up around that oppress LGBTQ people—and the voices that are for my greatest good and that uplift me.

Yoga helps me to constantly assess the damage that life has done to me and creates the space for me to be able to heal that damage.

Many times on the mat, the young boy that I was at various ages— the four-year-old playing in high-heeled boots on the porch, the insecure closeted gay adolescent in gym class, the fun-loving youth jumping double-dutch rope in the alley, the lonely, misfit, artsy, black, closeted gay teenager bravely navigating puberty—comes to me in my mind's eye and I wrap my grown-up arms around him and vow to become his hero. I have vowed to give him all the love and acceptance that he lacked growing up. I have vowed to tell him what the practice of yoga tells me every time I get on the mat: "You are enough!"

Yoga invites me to be my own hero. It's not a practice about comparing myself to other men. You don't have to do yoga how a man would do yoga. You don't have to do yoga like a woman would do yoga. You are invited to do yoga how YOU do yoga.

I am now living in a time when LGBTQ people are becoming more visible and more widely accepted. But, there are still many people who do not accept members of this marginalized group. The difference is that now I accept myself.

Through the practice of yoga, I am undoing the damage done to me so long ago that started with the teen yelling at me as I joyously played in women's high-heeled boots on the porch of my childhood home.

I am working on embracing the vision of what that grandfatherly man compassionately predicted way back in my elementary school gym class and what the black writers whose books I read as a teen wrote about. I am working on being a soldier that fights for my own personal freedom. I am working on being my own hero and basking in the light of my own glorious journey. I am working on healing and learning from my own traumatic history. I am working on telling my own story.

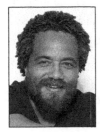

Dorian Christian Baucum was born in Washington, DC. His mission as a singer-songwriter is to create conscious music that people can groove to and events that help people get through life in a better way. He's the creator of Dorian's Live Neosoul & Yoga: a collaborative event that fuses his live music with yoga. He served in the Music for Healing program at Cedars-Sinai Medical Center and holds an MFA in acting from the University of California, San Diego. He's also a registered community pharmacist.

Author photo by David Young-Wolff.

# MOVEMENT OF AWAKENING

*Niralli Tara D'Costa*

Breath moves like waves through my body, casting circles through my hips, knees, shoulders, neck, and spine. The ocean swirls and crashes in the bay of my belly, my chest a sail full of wind. My jaw drops in ecstasy, and I feel the carpet-like sand beneath my feet. My head and my arms reach toward the pull of many directions. My hands engage in a dialogue with the cosmos, the ancestors, and celestial beings. They indicate what is happening inside of me: they listen and they hear.

I begin my movement practice by bringing awareness into my body, anchoring my legs into the ground. My mind focuses on the sensations of my body. My breath drops to meet them, creating patterns of expansion and contraction that draw my body into movement. I follow my impulses, which guide me deeper and deeper into my feeling awareness. The growing energy in my belly rises and expands into my upper body. My limbs awaken. My internal and external senses are present to the moments between moments and time is magnified. There is spaciousness within this state of being, which allows me to feel even more. All aspects of myself are safe here. My sorrow, my rage, my beauty, and my power are embodied in this dance.

My capacity for embodied experience comes from practicing a variety of movement modalities and receiving many forms of bodywork, and it stems from my lifelong practice of yoga and meditation. As an Indian woman, yoga was not something I "discovered," it was something that I grew up with; it was a thread in the fiber of daily life. I remember witnessing in curious silence while my grandmother meditated each day during her months' long visits from India. The energy would permeate the house, and as a child, I was free to participate or simply be in the space without interrupting. It was my grandmother who first taught me yogic postures and breath practices before I was old enough to read, and it was my family who taught me how to sit and listen and feel. They exposed me to the majesty of nature and the treasures of silence and deep listening.

It was also in my blood family that I would experience the trauma of childhood sexual abuse and the terror of domestic violence. It was these foundations of practice that gave me some sense of resource to come back to during unsettling times. In traditional tantric practice, the nectars and the poisons are both part of the alchemy that comprises the awakening process. So it was with my family: the nectars were given to transform and transmute the poisons that were presented to me there.

I met my first formal yoga teacher, Mansour, at the age of fourteen. He was visiting from India on a home exchange with the father of a dear friend. He taught me much about the nature of the mind and what it means to be a true yogi: to develop strength and flexibility not only of body but of mind, emotion, and energy. He was able to hold the depth and wisdom of the spiritual traditions he carried while meeting my fourteen-year-old level of maturity with humor and generosity.

For weeks he tried to teach my friend and me a pranayama practice called the breath of fire, which is a rapid series of forced exhales meant to raise heat in the body, and each time I would burst into laughter which would then cause my friend to start laughing.

Instead of scolding us or giving up, Mansour would join us in laughter week after week until eventually in class one day we didn't burst into laughter and were able to join him in the breath of fire practice. It was during these yoga sessions that I would learn about the possibility of opening into a space beyond my reactive mind and into a state of pure awareness. He taught us how to control the breath and work with our consciousness while practicing asana.

After our yoga sessions, he would often invite us to join him and his eight-year-old son for tea and toast. Watching him interact with his son was like watching a mountain transform into a babbling brook. Here this man who held such a vast body of knowledge and energetic capacity would turn into an innocent, giggling eight-year-old boy. He had this ability to fluidly join the energy of anyone he was interacting with, with the full potency and capacity of his enlightened heart. He was a true model of integration.

It was Mansour who initiated me into meditation with mantra. It was during that experience that I fully felt the reality of the nature of my physical form for the first time. I was only able to study with him for about a year before he went back home to India, but what he taught me through the practice, through his presence, and through his compassionate and open heart has given me an invaluable foundation as a practitioner ever since. It is a rare and precious blessing to encounter a yogi of his depth and level of awakening in today's world of commercialized spiritual culture.

About a year later, following a custody court battle, bearing witness to the cycle of domestic violence, escaping into drugs and alcohol, and uncovering repressed memories of childhood sexual abuse, I began studying yoga with Julian Walker. Julian had fled South Africa as a young anti-apartheid activist and musician, and he had begun his journey as a yoga practitioner before it was popular to do so.

I could relate to Julian's revolutionary spirit and independent spiritual impulse. At that time, I was practicing yoga for the purpose of building strength and flexibility, learning structural alignment, and for emotional and energetic purification. Julian was always inviting us to come back to our own personal experience on the mat, letting go of all the socially constructed rules of embodiment, and allowing yoga to be a space of hard work, release, and play. Practicing with Julian provided a solid ground during my tumultuous teenage and young adult years.

A couple of years into my studies with Julian, I began studying choreography and Gabrielle Roth's 5Rhythms with Michael Molin-Skelton. This allowed me to feel that I could safely access any emotion with the physical movements of my body as a vehicle. It was in his class, in the rhythm of chaos, that I was able to embody my repressed defenses against the sexual abuse that I suffered as a child. Pushing against the space of my embodied victimization, I was able to be present with, and be witnessed in, my trauma and rage. And it was in the rhythm of stillness that I was able to touch the deep despair of that wounded child, to feel how isolated and afraid she was while being held in the loving space of Michael's presence.

At that time, I began to experience large energetic and emotional releases in my yoga classes with Julian. I found my flexibility increasing at an intensified rate. The veil between my yogic practice and my perceptual reality became more and more translucent. Ecstatic, expressive dancing opened up this doorway for me in a way that it had not before because it gave me permission to fully participate in all aspects of my internal experience and a language to articulate that experience. In my work with Michael I could experience and process a full range of emotions without fear. This freedom translated into my yoga practice through the movement of energy guided by the breath in my body. Julian not only welcomed this in his classes but facilitated it beautifully. He constantly encouraged his students to focus on their internal experience, to follow the movement of energy, and to use the breath as a tool for release and expansion.

As more energy began to open up in my yoga practice, I became increasingly aware of the physical and energetic blockages that were present in my body. At that time, I began to receive trauma release bodywork from Julian. As I became a bodywork client of Julian's, I decided that I wanted to take my own work as a massage therapist and energy worker to the next level, so I trained in his Open Sky Bodywork. It was through this work that I was first introduced to the field and theories of somatic psychology, laying a foundation for my understanding of trauma's impact on the nervous system. As I grew in my understanding and worked with the principles of the modality, deeper and deeper layers of energetic and emotional release were happening in the bodywork sessions I received.

As a result, even more energy opened up in my body. I began to feel overwhelmed because I didn't know how to work with all of the energy available to me through my yoga practice, and I began to see the need for a more refined energetic practice. That is when I found Nita Rubio, teacher of The Tantric Dance of Feminine Power (TDFP). TDFP gave me the skills necessary to digest all of the energy that was awakening within me. I learned how to absorb and contain it while focusing my intention on self-love and divine connection. When I first came to this practice, experiencing pleasure was difficult for me. As a survivor of sexual abuse, I had learned to brace against pleasure. The Dance challenged me to be receptive to the pleasure inherent in surrendering to my own impulses with a devotional heart. Nita gently and skillfully guided me to reassociate with my bodily sensations by naming and appreciating what I was experiencing.

I learned that with spacious awareness all aspects of experience could be reintegrated into a sense of wholeness and that this process of integration is really what healing is all about. As I brought this new awareness to my practice as a bodyworker, my clients began unwinding trauma and experiencing deep emotional release during our sessions. I recognized that in order to practice responsibly, I needed to develop the skills necessary to help them make sense of what was happening and build coherence between their preexisting sense of themselves and the newly emerging experiences they were having. This is how I came to the formal study of Somatic Psychology at John F. Kennedy University's School of Holistic Studies. I was thrilled to have found a body of knowledge that provided a theoretical and scientific context for what I had been learning through my own experience of recovering from childhood trauma.

This knowledge empowered me to guide others in their own journeys of embodied healing as a holistic psychotherapist, and as my spiritual studies continued, I began linking the philosophical perspectives of Buddhism, tantra, and shamanism into the conceptual framework that I practiced therapy within. This included expanding perspectives from integration on the level of personal experience to include helping clients develop a relationship with the All That Is, that larger field of consciousness where everything is part of an even greater whole; to recognize their interrelatedness with all things and to witness their own mind and emotions.

I was finally ready, after a lifetime of knowing her, to study with one of my greatest teachers: my sister Gitanjali Hemp, visionary and founder of Syntara System, an innovative and profoundly integrative energy healing modality. Syntara System has allowed me to weave the energetic resources I've cultivated through my own spiritual practice into my therapeutic work seamlessly, in ways that are accessible to clients coming from a variety of spiritual perspectives and worldviews. This work allows me to facilitate coherence between vast cosmic fields of energy and clients' innermost embodied selves, allowing them to connect with spiritual nourishment via their felt sense and reorganize their mind, body, emotions, and identities in relationship with a deep sense of resource.

One of my greatest joys is to practice this work outdoors with clients. Leading experiential workshops and offering individual sessions amidst the living elements increases the energetic and embodied resources available and puts us in direct relationship with that greater whole. My studies with the Earthbody Institute gave me the practical skills and knowledge to take this leap. I feel so blessed that I am able to share with others what I have learned from my own healing journey and continue to learn and be transformed by the wisdom revealed in embodied therapeutic process.

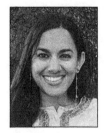

Niralli Tara D'Costa is a holistic psychotherapist LMFT (#54007), sacred embodiment teacher, and energy healer. She draws upon her long-term study of yoga, meditation, and tantra to support people on their spiritual path and healing journey. She is passionate about serving people who have traditionally been marginalized, as she sees social justice as central to our collective liberation, healing, and evolution. She currently serves as affiliate faculty in the Spiritual and Depth Psychology Department at Antioch University, and teaches in the Syntara System School of Energy Awareness as well as in the MindBody Therapy Certificate program in the online educational platform Embodied Philosophy. Read more about her work at nirallitara.com.

Author photo by Texas Isaiah.

# PART FOUR: REFLECTION QUESTIONS

- What practices will assist me in acknowledging my experiences of trauma while defining what they mean to me instead of being defined by them?
- What toxic thoughts and narratives am I ready to release?
- How am I allowing my practice of yoga to change me?
- If I deepen my love for myself ...?

—Michelle C. Johnson

# PART FIVE

## *Family and Belonging*

*Intergenerational trauma* is a term used to describe trauma that is passed down through communities and families from one generation to the next. Many of us are working to understand and heal the effects of intergenerational trauma as we navigate our way through life and attempt to forge identities of our own. Though yoga is by no means a cure-all or a substitute for professional care, the introspective nature of the practice can help us to ask important questions and define our core values by tapping into embodied wisdom. In this way, yoga can serve as a key ally and source of strength as we continuously and compassionately work to break cycles of trauma.

In her essay, "A Storied Family," Justine Mastin reflects on stories from her family's history, her journey toward yoga, and how her love of stories helped her to carve out a unique space in the yoga world, establishing a welcoming community for those who often do not feel welcome in yoga spaces.

Dr. Sará King shares her experience of chronic homelessness in childhood, how her relationship with her body reflected her experience, and how using her yoga practice as a means of self-expression helped her to reclaim a strong sense of embodiment and empowerment.

In "On the Yoga of Not Having a Baby," Kathleen Kraft explores expectations about gender roles and relationships and how her practice of yoga—which she describes as "a loyal friend"—helped her to connect with her intuition and confidently forge a path that honored her needs and nurtured her gifts.

For Elliot Kesse, therapy and yoga have played separate yet important roles in cultivating self-worth and healthy boundaries, helping them realize the important balance between self-growth and self-acceptance.

In her heartfelt narrative, Celisa Flores describes the role that yoga and meditation have played throughout her life, from being a small child practicing alongside her mother in a dimly lit church, to distancing herself from her practice as a young teenager who struggled with an eating disorder, to reconnecting with her body and practice during an unexpected pregnancy, to rediscovering the gifts of yoga again in adulthood. She explores yoga's role as a steady, healing constant in her life—a resource that helped her to cultivate community and resilience and, ultimately, to share those gifts with others.

Antesa Jensen shares a raw, deeply personal essay about the effects of childhood trauma on her relationship to her body and self-image. She explains how a yoga practice that initially began as another means of achieving "perfection" helped her to establish an appreciation for her body's innate wisdom, paving the way for the work that would lead to a healthier relationship with herself and others.

Similarly, yoga coupled with therapy allowed Sanaz Yaghmai to reattune to a strong mind-body connection, which helped her confidently subvert cultural and familial expectations and heal from physical and emotional trauma. In "The Alchemy of Trauma," she explains that, while as a therapist she understood this connection intellectually, it was the embodied experience of her practice that helped her to fully reap its benefits, helping her to feel at home in her body.

# MEDITATION

## *Coming Home to Embodied Presence*

We will start with a breathing practice to quiet your mind.

Find a comfortable seat or, if you prefer, you can stand or lie down. To find a comfortable seat you might want to elevate your hips by sitting on a cushion, pillow, or blanket.

Close your eyes or look at the ground in front of you and begin to breathe into your body. Start by taking deep breaths in and out. Begin to feel the shape change in your body as you breathe. Notice the expansion as you inhale and the contraction or release with your exhale.

Notice any sensations and emotions.

As you breathe, visualize an image that represents returning home to your center and core of who you truly are. This might be an image of a physical structure that represents home or a cycle of breath to bring you back to center. You might visualize a person, landscape, or being. Visualize something or someone that represents coming home to the center and core of who you truly are. Notice everything you can about this image—the colors, sounds, scents, and feelings you experience when you return home.

Be with this image for a few minutes.

If you want to connect a mantra with your image you can repeat the words "So Hum," which means, "I am that" or "Thou art that."

You are this image of home; you can return to your core and who you truly are at any time. This image came from you and represents you.

If you want to work the mantra, repeat "So Hum" three times.

Once you feel ready to move out of this meditation, return to the breath. Return to the expansion and contraction, emotions and sensations.

As you feel ready, gently open your eyes or lift your gaze and re-orient to the space around you. Notice any colors, sounds, or familiar sights in the space. Take a moment to remember you are home. Home is within you. It is always available to you.

—Michelle C. Johnson

# A STORIED FAMILY

## Justine Mastin

My legacy is one of trauma. My mother passed it down to me from her mother, who received it from her mother, who no doubt received it from her mother and on and on. It is a legacy of scarcity and war and intolerance. My maternal grandmother was born in a Jewish shtetl in Hungary with three siblings, one of whom would never be spoken of—an uncle my mother didn't even know she had until adulthood. I would later learn that there were other family members who had been cut off due to some perceived wrong. Even without knowing, I knew that it was possible to be *abandoned*, which to my young brain meant *forgotten*. I knew that there could come a time when people would stop telling your story.

On the outside my family looked happy, and there were many ways in which we were—especially in our shared love of story and whimsy—but I knew that something didn't feel right. It was confusing because there wasn't something to immediately point to and say, "That's what's wrong." At the time I didn't know that this *something* was inherited trauma. Most people are familiar with the concept of trauma, but the concept of transgenerational (or intergenerational) trauma may be new for many. When we speak of transgenerational trauma, we speak of the ways that an individual or group passes down both the story and the emotional pain of a lived event to subsequent generations. As children, we pick up on the subtlest cues from our primary caregivers. Through both their genes and their affect, my parents passed on their families' trauma to me. My experience is hardly unique because "[c]hildren are constantly observing their parents' gestures and affects, absorbing their parents' conscious and unconscious minds … This is how stories are told, even when not spoken, in the nonverbal and preverbal affective realms—silent and vocal, yet played out in subtexts, often on the implicit level."[35]

The cut-offs in my mother's family baffled me as a young person. How could someone simply be removed from a family? As an adult, and especially as a psychotherapist, I am aware that there was nobody to model relationship repair for my mother. The lesson that she learned was that repair is impossible and the only answer is estrangement. At the time, however, the message that I received was simply this: people can be forgotten. Yet I was terrified to be truly seen because the real me might not be acceptable and I would still be pushed away. It was a catch-22.

## Anxiety

I was a dancer and actor, appearing on the stage, where no one could deny that I existed, where I could not be forgotten. And yet I still felt invisible, like a ghost that was walking among the living. Never fully embodying myself, always just slightly apart on the other side of the veil. What I showed to the world was not the full me, more of an echo of me. I realized the function of my behavior only decades after the fact: I was so desperate to be seen, to not be one of the forgotten, that the stress of this grasping to be noticed manifested in a profound anxiety. Anxiety became my constant companion—at least I wasn't suffering alone.

I suffered through my anxiety, pushed past my discomfort daily, because the pain of not being seen was worse than the pain of living that

35. Jill Salberg, "The Texture of Traumatic Attachment: Presence and Ghostly Absence in Transgenerational Transmission," *The Psychoanalytic Quarterly* 84, no. 1 (January 2015): 21–46, https://doi.org/10.1002/j.2167-4086.2015.00002.x.

life, and this behavior was supported, even nurtured. The night before my first day of work waiting tables at age seventeen, in an attempt to assuage my nerves, my father said, "Just act like a server." *Yes, acting*, I thought, *I know how to do that*.

The greatest respite from my constant anxiety was engaging with stories: watching television and movies in particular. I imagined myself a part of those worlds, somewhere else where maybe I could be me. I didn't show anyone in this world the real me for fear that if they met *that* person, the full authentic me (if I could even find her), that she would be unacceptable and be cut off like my great-uncle and others whom maybe I hadn't even heard of but whose absence I felt.

## Practice

I first stepped on a yoga mat as a child in the 1980s. I attended a class with my mother, and I couldn't stand it—the slowness of it. I longed for the torturous movement of my dance classes. The quiet and stillness gave me too much space to think and to be alone with my anxiety. But I remained curious about the possibilities of yoga asana, particularly about the yogis who seemed so calm and so obviously authentic (I assumed). Over time I would return to my practice, through a book that I found in my mother's room that offered a bit of peace to an angsty high schooler, and again in college for a physical education credit.

My practice finally stuck in my early twenties when I discovered a power vinyasa and hot yoga practice. I loved the movement, the sweating, the way that my body somehow felt both challenged and loved. And it helped my anxiety. I was able to discharge the energy that was built up inside of me. The hardest part was getting myself to go. The anticipatory distress was sometimes too much to get me into my stretchy pants. Even though the yoga itself was healing, the atmosphere was not. I felt like I had to put on a show just like I did everywhere else in my life. I looked the part of these other yoga practitioners, but I didn't feel like them. Those yogis, who I'd assumed were so calm and authentic from afar, felt like they were judging me up close. But I knew that the physical practice helped because I could feel it in my body and so I kept going back and *acting* like a yogi. There were now two places where I could get a respite from my anxiety—in stories and on the mat.

## Loss

I began seriously working with a therapist in my late twenties and committed to my healing with my entire self. I suffered through every painful assignment. I see a similar suffering on the faces of my own clients, a suffering that I can't take away from them because the process of moving through their suffering is how they will heal.

About a year into my therapy journey, my father passed away suddenly. He'd dealt with health problems for many years, but he'd always bounced back. His desire to stay in the spotlight always drew him away from that metaphorical bright light. This time it didn't. The grief of losing my father, and right as I was beginning this new understanding of myself, was unbearable. But as so often happens with grief, it was also the catalyst to explore my own life. I decided that I wasn't satisfied with how I was living—on the outside looking in. Operating out of fear, the fear of being forgotten. Simply begging to be seen but not truly allowing anyone to see me for fear that if they saw me, they would retreat.

I decided that I would change what my life looked like, that I would move from a career in the "administrative arts" to one focused on well-being. I was and am fortunate to have the privilege to do this: both systemic privilege and a supportive partner provided me with the emotional and financial safety nets that enabled this shift. It was New Year's Eve 2009, three months after my father's passing and a million feelings later, that I committed to sign up for yoga teacher training and apply to graduate school. I was opening myself up to being seen, for real this time. I was going to allow people to see the authentic me rather than the created self whom I shared for so long. At least that's what I thought.

## Training

I did my yoga teacher training with one of the "big box" yoga studios where I had been practicing. Even though I didn't feel totally comfortable there, I didn't feel totally comfortable anywhere, and this is where my yoga asana journey had flourished. My cohort was huge, more than fifty people—a serious contrast to the teacher trainings that I later led and capped at six people. But this large group offered some sense of security because I wouldn't be seen too much too early. How could I be? I was able to slip through unnoticed until the day that we practiced teaching to the entire cohort instead of our usual small groups.

I taught tree pose, and while we were given a strict script for how to guide it, I ad-libbed that the group was "such a beautiful forest of trees." I sat down and awaited my feedback given in the form of roses (for positive feedback) and thorns (for challenges). The first words out of the lead trainer's mouth were "I've never heard you talk that much before." I didn't hear anything after that. The roses and thorns were lost as I experienced my own catharsis. Tears were uncontrollably flowing down my cheeks. I was vaguely aware that everyone was staring at me, that they likely thought I was upset about my feedback, which I wasn't aware of at all.

As soon as they'd finished showering me with roses and thorns, I ran out of the room and hid in the bathroom to cry. To be alone with the enormity of what had just happened. The vulnerability that I'd just experienced. I was aware that the co-lead trainer had come into the bathroom to look for me, but I continued to hide. Eventually I did go back in and finish the day, and at the end, the co-trainer pulled me aside. I was embarrassed, thinking that I was going to have to explain what happened and that yes, "I'm ok." But she just said, "I see you." I was shocked. My words tumbled out in a torrent, hurriedly explaining that I wasn't upset about the feedback, that it was just so much being vulnerable like that, being so visible, and she said, "I know." I had been seen. I had been understood. I thanked that teacher at the time for those words and followed up later to let her know just how much they meant to me. They still do.

It was both a small and a hugely profound moment that was transformative. It took hundreds of hours of my own work—on and off the mat—and the guidance of a skilled therapist to get there, for me to let that moment happen, for me to let it in. And the fear I'd had of going to grad school suddenly felt lessened. If I could be seen like this, if I could show up for people on the mat, then maybe I could show up for people off the mat as well. Maybe I could even show up for myself.

## Frustration

But of course, this isn't the end of the story. Sometimes stories end there with the transformation and the realization and the happily ever after. But this transformation is a process that you live, a process that I lived and I still live. Generations of trauma that were passed on to me did not simply release and free me, but there was a small crack in my defensive armor. Even after feeling seen, I still wasn't totally comfortable showing my authentic self. The feedback that I received in subsequent reviews was that I wasn't being authentic, that I was using a "yoga teacher" voice. *Well, of course I am*, I thought. Remembering back to what my father had said, "just act" like a yoga teacher. I was still acting. Even as I tried to tap into my authentic self, I kept bumping up against something. And that something was the system I was trying to inhabit. I could not be myself within this system that I didn't believe in. I didn't believe in up-selling yoga mats or giving hands-on adjustments to people who hadn't asked for them. It isn't that yoga didn't fit; *this* yoga didn't fit. I needed to stop acting *as if* and instead start embodying my work and my life.

## Introspection

I turned inward to ask myself what was missing, and the answer was that I was ignoring an entire part of myself. The part of me that was filled up by stories had been ignored. And so that summer I attended my first comic con. Another pivotal turning point in my life was just on the horizon. I loved being around other folks who loved stories in the same way that I did. I felt at home. As I looked around at all of those kindred spirits, outsiders like me that the world derogatorily called geeks, I wondered who was looking out for them; who was helping them to care for themselves when the rest of the world saw them as one of the few groups that it was still acceptable to openly shame? And in that moment, I made a commitment to create a style of yoga that didn't just welcome the outsider but was created for them, for their benefit, healing, and longevity. In that moment, what would become YogaQuest, a narrative style of yoga, was born.

## Bravery

I took a flying leap into the water of authenticity. I created a yoga class that linked together asana with the narratives that I loved. I stood up in front of a room and presented this thing that I had made. I had created something that came from within me using the two aspects that had helped me through some of my own darkest times. I let myself be seen without a mask and allowed the chips to fall where they may. I knew in that moment that this strange hybrid creature I'd created could be an abomination that would take one gasp and then die, but that isn't what happened. My strange creation was met with joy and wonder, and by the time she was met with criticism, I loved her so much that it didn't matter. I put myself into the narrative of my own life and the story was sweeter than I ever could have imagined. Now *this* is my legacy. Trauma shaped me and the way that I see the word—stories and yoga changed me, and I changed them.

Mantra: I am a living, breathing story, telling itself.

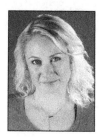

Justine Mastin, MA, LMFT, LADC, E-RYT 200, YACEP, is the owner and founder of Blue Box Counseling & Wellness and the fearless leader of Yoga-Quest. She has contributed to a number of pop culture and psychology books and is the captain of the *Starship Therapise* podcast. Justine takes a holistic approach to healing: mind, body, and fandom. Visit her online at blueboxcounseling.com.

Author photo by Markei Photo & Video.

# ON YOGA AND CHRONIC HOMELESSNESS: A MEDITATION

*Dr. Sará King*

It is probably fairly commonplace for mothers to have conversations with their children about their birth story. I know I have recounted the story of my daughter's birth to her time and time again. She listens to it with deep fascination and glee, this retelling of her very first moments in the world. My recollection always starts with the moment where she emerged from my body into a birthing tub—me standing up and literally roaring like a Mother Bear—into this beautiful, strange, and chaotic place that would be her new home so long as she should be blessed to live. I imagine that children all over the world ask lots of questions about their birth story—such as where exactly were they born, was it a long or short labor, what did the mama first recall about how she felt when she laid eyes on her child's face for the very first time? The story of my birth, as told to me by my own mother, goes a little something like this:

She, a single African American woman alone in a hospital room in a lonely California farm town. The doctors, all white and male, and in a considerably different position of power then she, come barging into the delivery room and insist on inducing her labor so I would come out faster. She resists against their dominating pleas, even going so far as to waddle out into the hallway and lie down on the ground where she can be away from their prying eyes and escalating demands. Moments after getting her body onto the ground, the contractions start coming extremely quickly, and out I come, slipping and sliding onto the glaringly white hospital floor. The doctors find her there and are alarmed—they grab me from her arms to see if I am breathing yet. I am not. Little infant Sará (me) is looking slightly blue in the face, and time is running out to get me to give the proper physiological breathing response. My mother worriedly looks on as one doctor decides to try a noninvasive approach.

Supposedly, I was curled into a little ball, my arms crossed over each other on my chest, and my legs were wrapped around one another as well. In my mind's eye, I pictured a sweet little brown-skinned baby, legs in eagle pose, and arms wrapped in a "give-yourself-a-hug" asana. Which totally makes sense. I imagined that even coming out of the womb, my body knew which pose to take to express self-love and my protective instincts. The attending doctor put my body in one of his hands, my back against his palm, and raised me abruptly into the air. Apparently, as the story goes, the shock of this change in my sense of equilibrium caused me to open up my arms wide into a capital letter T shape, my legs splayed straight and about hip width apart. But instead of screaming or crying out loud as many newborn babies did, I opened my mouth and took one great big, hearty, audible sigh... and then I returned to my previous pose, arms hugged about my body tight, legs wrapped in eagle once again. Except this time around, I continued to gently breathe.

I laugh and smile to myself whenever I think about my birth story today, because for one thing, it is the story of one of my mother's frequent Afro-feminist political protests against enduringly white institutions that have sought to take control of her body and her life. My mother was a staunch advocate for civil rights her entire life. At one point having been a member of the Black Panther party, she put her life and limb on the line for the freedoms that I enjoy to this day. The other thing that strikes me about my birth story is that, to me, it is also the story of my very first yoga practice in this world. My practice may have only been three asanas long, but the fact that my body knew instinctively, through its somatic intelligence, that panicking and screaming would not produce a calm nervous system response to help orient myself to just having come into this world, never ceases to amaze me. My body knew that breathing in deep and embracing myself with love was an appropriately soothing response to the shock of all of the new embodied sensations I was feeling. In retrospect, my birth story is deeply indicative of the path that my life would take in my journey back home to myself.

## Searching for Solid Ground: On Pain and Invisibility

I find it interesting how much easier it was for me to see challenges as opportunities to play when I was a child. Perhaps it was because I had not seen enough of the world to feel jaded or completely mistrusting of it yet. By the time I was nine years old, I had already lived in far too many apartments and motel rooms to count. Though I did not know it at the time, my mother was struggling with a variety of different untreated mental illnesses that made it incredibly difficult for her to hold down a stable job. That, and the fact that she was born in the body of a very beautiful, dark-skinned, voluptuous woman, who had not (for a variety of political reasons) been able to finish her college degree, meant that she faced an endless, Sisyphean mountain of racism and sexism that resulted in younger white women getting hired for virtually every single secretarial job that she applied for.

We developed a habit of moving to a new town, sometimes in a new state, every two to three months. She would apply for apartments, and upon getting into one and paying for the first month's rent, we knew that the landlord technically had sixty to ninety days before she or he would call the sheriff's office and have us forcibly removed. Together, we would fashion makeshift desks for us to read and do work on out of two-by-four planks of wood and plastic crates acquired at the local Home Depot—I got more splinters than you can possibly imagine getting my homework done! An egg carton mattress topper, no more than an inch thick, would serve as our beds. I was so used to sleeping on them that by the time I was fourteen and finally slept in a real bed, I would sometimes sleep on the ground still because I couldn't get used to the softness of a mattress.

Inevitably, the landlord would start sending home threatening letters, and we knew that we would have to be on the run again. We would flee from the apartment, sometimes with only a few hours' notice, the police on our heels. She would only allow me to take a few articles of clothing with me. Everything and anything else I had acquired, which wasn't much—maybe a few stuffed animals and my school things— would get tossed without fanfare into a nearby dumpster. On we would move into a motel room in another city, or sometimes into the back of a U-Haul truck that she would rent using an alias, effectively highjacking the truck from the establishment that she had hoodwinked into thinking we would pay for it. The two of us would cuddle up together and sleep on the metal floor of the truck, shivering through the night. We more often than not had barely anything to eat, subsisting on bread, cheese, and lentils. Wherever we ended up, she would apply for welfare so we would have enough money to tide us over for a little something to eat. Our family on the opposite coast from us, hearing about our destitution, would invariably send us money so that we could at least get into an apartment and out of an endless string of motels and other welfare housing.

This endless rotating in and out of homes, and in and out of schools as well, with mostly nothing but the clothes on my back, seemed to drag on forever. Though I was often terrified of where we would end up next, I think I tried to maintain a positive attitude and look at us as adventurous vagabonds on the run. Anywhere we went, I remember gazing out of the window of some public bus, eyeballing houses and apartments and wondering what it would be like to actually have a steady home.

During the day, my mother would oftentimes leave me alone at a battered women's shelter that we called our temporary home, in a local library, or at a bus stop near the shelter to wait for her to return. I never knew how long it would take her to come home, whether she was looking for a job, or what in the world she was doing. At this point in my story I am ten years old. I remember one day, while waiting at a bus stop all alone for hours on end, there was an older African American man lying in the gutter in mud spattered, torn clothing some hundred paces away from me. He appeared to me to be in some kind of drug-induced reverie, but he was covered in sores and moaning loudly as though he was in the very last throes of his life. Then he started shaking and went completely still. He laid there not moving for the next five hours while I waited for my mother to come back. In that moment, two things happened. I began to contemplate the likelihood that my life would end in the same way: alone, shivering, and writhing in pain somewhere in a city gutter with no one to know that I was gone. The second thing that happened was I started to consciously diminish my breath. Somehow, it occurred to me that I could slow my breath down to barely a trickle, my chest beginning to concave and my shoulders hunching forward, and this manner of breathing seemed to reflect everything I was feeling inside. Breathing like this made me feel like I was barely alive, and I wanted to feel that way. Though I had suicidal thoughts throughout my childhood, this was my first attempt at making myself invisible. I figured that maybe eventually I would stop breathing altogether just like that man, and death would bring me release from the incredible emotional and physical pain that made my body feel like a trap.

This physiological response, I realize today, represented the opposite of my body's deepest intuitive inclination, which is to lean into life using the healing power of the breath, as I knew how to even during the process of my birth. By the age of ten, I had learned to replace my life instinct with a death instinct. Though I did not have the wherewithal to end my life outright, I was determined to restrict my functioning in the world and my ability to be seen—lest I be targeted by some awful form of violence. I thought that maybe by barely breathing, I might slip under the radar of all of the predators of life, numb and invisible not only to the world, but to myself. It was the only game plan that I had; that, and somehow managing to consistently shock and awe my teachers with my ability to ace all of my schoolwork in spite of my bedraggled and clearly malnourished appearance.

Something deep down inside of me must have known that living this life was worth it for me to continue to survive and thrive academically in spite of my daunting circumstances. The rest of my story, from age ten to seventeen when I was finally accepted into some of this nation's best colleges—with a full scholarship no less—is far too much to tell in the span of this chapter. I will say that when I was thirteen years old, my mother, who had been physically abusing me throughout our relationship, offered me the chance to move with her to Canada or threatened to leave me by myself to face the world. I had run away from her several times by that point, fighting for my life, only to be returned to her by the police. I chose to be homeless, this time on my own, and let her leave to pursue her own destiny.

I was incredibly lucky to have friends who found out about my situation and let me live in their homes temporarily until my extended family took me in for the rest of my high school years. Without their help, I may have endured a fate worse than the man by the bus stop. As a little girl constantly abandoned and left to my own devices in the streets, it is truly a miracle that I didn't end up sex trafficked or in jail. For years, I continued to hold my breath painfully, my muscles wracked with the ever-present memory of the trauma of chronic homelessness, malnourishment, and neglect, among other abuses that my body had survived up until that point. It wasn't until after college, at the age of twenty-one, that I rediscovered the healing power of my breath, and indeed how to live my life and express myself fully again through the practice of yoga.

## How to House the Soul: The Journey Back Home Again

When I began my yoga practice at the age of twenty-one, it felt like everything in my body was on fire. My lungs screamed when I took in a deep breath; I absolutely could not fathom how anyone could aspire to the "one-breath-per-asana" description that was so breezily instructed by my yoga teachers. I wanted to pass out halfway through class. I usually spent the last thirty minutes in child's pose, crying gently onto my mat and trying not to curl into a fetal position. I absolutely hated it.

I not-so-secretly glared at all of the svelte yoga bodies all around me, looking so limber and flexible and glowing like they didn't have a care in the world. Most of the people in the classes that I took seemed to be young, blond, skinny, and far more moneyed than I was. I winced visibly at the sight of signs advertising twenty dollars per class; it was about a fifth of my food budget for the week. Identifying myself as a "yogi," as some instructors called us, seemed about as far off a possibility as me becoming an astronaut and actually going to Mars. I tried to convince myself that the practice wasn't for me and to abandon it altogether.

As a last ditch effort to keep up with the practice and avoid the shame I felt inside of yoga studios, I decided to buy a yoga DVD and practice in the comfort of my own home where my comparative mind wouldn't drive me crazy trying to look like everyone else. The DVD was by Shiva Rea, and she didn't look anything like me, a young African American woman, but there was something about her countenance, her visible joy, and tone of voice that was comforting and spoke to me of the possibility of peace. I soldiered on, starting out with fifteen- to twenty-minute practices that left me winded and inevitably crying somewhere on my bedroom floor. I just didn't understand why it hurt so much—especially the breathing part! During the practice I felt like I was experiencing a living hell. But what kept me coming back was the savasana, the period of rest at the very end. Each time I lay there in complete stillness after a yoga practice, a calm descended on me that was completely transformative. Though the savasana was only five minutes out of my day, in that time, my breathing started to return to something of what I remembered from the earliest years of my childhood, when I knew how to express myself freely and nothing held me back from the feeling of self-love. What I didn't realize until years into my practice was that I was slowly returning home, but this time, the discovery of home was within my own body. Eight years into my practice, I had the great fortune to attend a yearlong yoga and meditation teacher training at Spirit Rock, and the eminent yogi Rolf Gates was one of my fellow trainees. When I told him about my experience with homelessness earlier on in life, he invited me to see how my practice might shift if I invoked the feeling of being home in downward dog by concentrating on the connection between my feet and the earth. My practice has literally never been the same ever since. Now, the simple act of walking while placing my awareness in my feet brings me back to a potent feeling of returning home. My practice over time has slowly shifted from an agonizing chore to a rejuvenating dance of self-love and remembrance that brings me time and time again to the felt experience of liberation and home inside of myself.

It has now been nearly fifteen years since I first started my yoga practice, and learning to love it was definitely not easy. Perhaps it is not the yoga that was challenging to learn to love, but rather, it was the journey to loving myself again after so many years of living in survival mode and accumulating self-hatred that was very hard to heal within my body. I have practiced yoga on four different continents, in dozens of studios, and in every home I have lived in since. It has carried me with grace and supported my resilience through all of the ups and downs that life has had to bring. One thing is for certain. Nowadays, when I take a series of deep breaths and hug myself while I am on my mat (as I am often prone to do), I am reminded that my body's somatic intelligence knew what home felt like since I took my very first breath. I needed no instructor— heck, I didn't even need a stable roof over my head. Home is right here, in this body, in this present moment. It is available to me anytime I focus in and become aware of my breath. It doesn't need to arrive through a fancy pose or in a lushly appointed studio. Home is the compassionate, empowering feeling that radiates out from my cells and from my soul, reminding me to love, accept, and celebrate myself for exactly who I am—and that is a feeling that no one can take away from me.

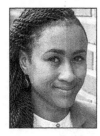

Sará King, PhD is a mother, a social and behavioral neuroscientist, medical anthropologist, political scientist, and an educator by training. As a translational research scientist at OHSU, she is developing culturally relevant ways to integrate mindfulness and yoga into cognitive and brain health based interventions for Alzheimer's prevention, as well as investigating the relationship between sleep behavior, pain, and perceived discrimination. She is also the creator of the "Science of Social Justice," a contemplative and evidence-based framework for scientific research and workshop facilitation dedicated to healing the dis-ease of "othering" and uplifting marginalized communities. Learn more about her work at mindheartconsulting.com.

Author photo by Kelly Erickson Craft Media Solutions.

# ON THE YOGA OF NOT HAVING A BABY

## Kathleen Kraft

I was forty and teaching creative movement and yoga at an elementary school to first through fourth graders. I started working at the school in my thirties after a series of personal and professional missteps, by which I mean choices I made that didn't ultimately serve me. Teaching there was the beginning of a new journey. But after a couple of years, it began to sink in that everyone around me was having babies. Young moms of my students were becoming moms *again*, my colleagues were going on maternity leave, friends were getting pregnant or adopting. I'd always wanted children; where were mine? Finally, I met someone I thought was the right person; we got engaged, we tried for a baby—faintheartedly on his part—and two years later we split up.

That is, of course, the short story.

So there I was, still teaching kids—bereft. What was once a beautiful job was becoming a chore; it was time to move on.

I carved a plan: I would move to a less expensive state (I'd been living and working in New Jersey and New York), and I'd look for a job teaching high school English (I had an MFA, had taught high school poetry, and worked as a dot-com editor), and I would adopt a child. That was the plan. I sent my application to the adoption agency.

And then I started practicing yoga regularly, intentionally. And slowly everything changed.

How do we become who we become? My life has been a series of organic openings. As soon as I chart a path, a new one begins to open, and I'm drawn toward it. But since I started practicing yoga, I've been able to follow my intuition more skillfully, connecting with parts of myself that have been dormant for a long time. They are no longer in conflict with one another, and I now have a deepening sense of, and respect for, my own nature. The process continues to evolve every day, often in surprising ways. Yoga has proven to be a loyal friend.

Before the practice took hold, I compared myself to others. Before yoga, I didn't *really* know I was comparing myself to others. I wasn't aware of the impact of my thoughts; they just happened. Before yoga, my life was a series of compartmentalized moves. And I grasped. A lot.

So there I was, in Jersey City, recently "disengaged," holed up with an iPad full of Netflix and diligently plotting out the rest of my life between episodes of *Lie to Me*. That's when I knew something had to change. I had a yoga mat—I'd been an off and on again practitioner— so I started practicing at the studio around the corner. I got lucky—it was spare and pretty, a space to take a break from all my turbulence. It was old school, too: a card catalogue system instead of MINDBODY®, a third floor walk-up that was occasionally locked when I got there early, a few carefully tended orchids, translucent white curtains, and a sweet little sitting area with small benches where students waited in between classes and whispered. And best of all, first-rate teachers.

I could literally move into a quieter, less judgmental reflection there. The breakup wasn't my first failed relationship. I'd been married once upon a time ago, and I'd gotten pregnant accidentally right before we got married. I terminated the pregnancy, a decision that still feels complicated even though I still believe it was the best one to make at the time. And although I terminated the marriage, I was in shambles after the breakup. Depressed and sleepless, I solved the problem with prescription medicine, and within a year I was back on my feet. Sort of. I now see that most of the coping mechanisms I had before yoga were temporary ones; they were solution, not process, oriented. My approach to psychotherapy was "When will I get better?"

Hatha and Anusara, with the occasional vinyasa flourish, was the style offered at my studio around the corner. Each teacher offered their own practice—you could feel that, and I'm not sure I've felt it that clearly anywhere else to date. The classes were never too big, and there were only two a day, not too many to choose from! I was there most days for about a year. It was my nourishment, a way to express myself outside of writing, which now felt too lonely to do regularly. I'd always loved dance and movement; teaching creative movement to young children fulfilled my need to experiment with different forms and create in the context of teaching, but I was searching for a real practice of my own. And moving on my mat in my home around the corner opened me up to my creativity in a new way. As a writer, the versatility and organization of the practice resonated with me.

Much has been written about the transformative quality of yoga, how it brings a practitioner into a greater, deeper experience of themselves. Part of this—perhaps especially for people who enjoy words and language—has to do with the subtle psychological effects of climbing inside the different personas the poses offer. We are warriors, moons, trees, snakes, suns … mountains. We are sages briefly. Abstract and specific, we can locate ourselves among these personas. In short, we play in a universe on our mats, one we create again and again.

And I was becoming strong. I felt good in my body. There was a new lightness that was easier—a freer way to perceive the world. Some of the teachers told stories—about Ganesh, about Hanuman. I sat there like one of my young students, rapt. I felt like a creature who could leap a great distance, and yet I had no idea where I was going. Wasn't I going to move to the country and raise a child?

This is hard to write. I'm not sure I'll ever make "complete peace" with not being a mother. And perhaps one day my situation will change and I'll foster a child. Lately, more existential concerns have risen up: I will have no legacy. The end of the gene pool. And so on.

I do have one nephew, whom I am incredibly grateful for.

But my yoga path took me in a different direction. I wanted to become a teacher. I wanted to teach yoga and movement to adults, and I knew that choosing that path would not be sustainable in the long-term in terms of raising a child. Maybe I would meet someone to share the responsibility with, but maybe I wouldn't while living out in the country. Ultimately, I chose yoga because more than having a child, I wanted to continue to delve into my own mystery.

I've heard yoga described as an ocean. As a poet, this metaphor has a healing effect on me. Yoga was a place where I could swim through poses, through philosophy, through chanting, through chakras, and so on. I could alight on the topic of reciprocal inhibition (the way muscles on one side of a joint contract in order to release on the other side of that joint) and then dip into the meaning of *sthira* (one of the essential qualities in a yoga pose, according to Patanjali; it means steady.) and *sukha* (the other essential quality, meaning comfortable) and let the connections between the two form. I did not have to force myself to learn yoga. Yoga learned me in an associative way. I could stop eating meat and I could start again; both made sense. I could feel the excitement and propulsion of vinyasa alongside the very different need for yin in my life. There was the beautiful coral reef of ayurveda to meander around. Once I completed my 200 hours, I continued my studies and pursued more certifications. I worked with several populations, including patients in a long-term rehab. Yoga became my moving poetry.

The passage below is from a blog post called "Teaching the Forgotten" I wrote in 2014 about teaching at the rehab. It illustrated yoga's impact on my consciousness and the way it connected me, personally, to the vulnerability of being alive: "One of the residents who attends my class wears a bib and doesn't move very much, but his eyes light up from time to time, and when I encourage him, he responds. Most are elderly women, over seventy-five, in wheelchairs. Most say little. Most look very tired. Michael uses a walker and is fighting; lines of pain and determination streak his face. He says I work them hard and thanks me. A woman named Sandra complains, "I don't like yoga," but she likes to wear the Chinese jump ropes I bring in (for stretching) around her neck.

This is my yoga. Teaching chair yoga at the rehab feeds me on a different level. On Tuesday mornings when I walk over, I feel as though I am walking toward the divine. Teaching has always felt like a spiritual act, but the care center is where I experience the feeling most directly."[36]

The care center was also a place where I found myself wondering why I was "taking care" of the elderly—again, where were my kids? At times I wonder if not having a child is connected in some way to fear, a fear of dying that possibly dates back to worrying about being orphaned. Fear works in complex ways and is quite possibly encoded in our DNA, according to recent research.[37] I am the granddaughter of a Jewish immigrant who hid in his parents' basement for months during the pogroms before escaping Russia and moving to the United States. How his fear was passed down to my mother and then to me, specifically, is something I've become more aware of over the years, a kind of living fear. One that hasn't necessarily prevented me from doing bold, adventurous things, but a fear that nonetheless seems to be a part of me. The part of me that needs to lock the door and check it again sometimes. The part that skims political headlines warily. My blood pressure rises when I learn about mass shootings. All of these reactions are, of course, understandable and probably relatable for many people.

But other things have happened. One of my high school teachers, who had a profound impact on me, was violently killed. This happened a few months after the elementary school shootings in Newtown, Connecticut, and after a longtime, respected teacher at my school was arrested (and later sentenced) for distributing child pornography online. I'll never forget those days. We were all still reeling from the aftermath of Hurricane Sandy, which had damaged the school and my neighborhood. It's hard to blow past facts that are staring all of us in the eye: population growth and inequality are factors in climate change; we, the global we, are having trouble feeding our children; there is a gun

36. Kathleen Kraft, "Teaching the Forgotten," Yogacity NY, November 16, 2014 https://yogacitynyc.wordpress.com/2014/11/16/teaching-the-forgotten/.

37. Martha Henriques, "Can the Legacy of Trauma be Passed Down the Generations?" BBC Future, BBC, March 26, 2019, https://www.bbc.com/future /article/20190326-what-is-epigenetics.

crisis. What I've grown to understand is that the longer I've waited to have children, the more the weight of the world and memory has impacted me. There *is* something to having kids when you're younger, less haunted, more idealistic—not thinking about how realistic it is to bring children into a world so fraught with unrest.

So, it was good to "take care" of these older people, to be a source of strength for them. And teaching still is a gratifying and *nurturing* experience for me: being able to help a student settle into their skin a little more, offering a delicious stretch that people can easily do at home, being able to place my hands lightly on shoulders at the end of class to help folks settle into rest more easily—these are the reasons I teach. But yoga naturally led me back to writing and editing, this time for yoga publications. I now feel most at home in yoga in this context: helping people who write about it clarify their vision and express themselves to their fullest. I like making their pieces sparkle—it's a privilege, one I may not have had if I had become a single mother. I most likely would've had to make less-fulfilling choices, and even in the gratifying context of being a mother, I imagine that would have been exceptionally difficult.

And I get to write about topics that are dear to my heart: making yoga accessible, yoga and social justice, employing poetry in the yoga space and, on occasion, poems about my own experience in movement. I like being a part of a bigger yoga family who is devoted to sharing the practice around the world. It gives me faith.

I also love what's happening in yoga, in particular the way functional movement and movement in general is beginning to loosen up the oft "tight joint space" of the practice, moving it in a more fluid direction. I now have an appreciation of my own creative movement explorations and a desire to share them with others. There is much to be grateful for in our yoga world; we can enjoy a childlike energy together if we let ourselves dive into the sea, float on the waves.

But what has yoga taught me about relationships? What have I learned about the mistakes I've made? I wish I could answer that easily.

Learning to trust my instincts is at the top of the list. In other words, making *embodied decisions*. Being able to carry my ease into a relationship. To be loved and to be able to give love more easily, without dragging my suitcase of past disappointments into it. To flow and then settle as you would in a supported posture.

Maybe the key is to find someone whose neurosis is familiar, one with whom your neuroses dovetail well. After all, if there's no rhythm, there's no dance. But I also know that in order to dance I need to feel good about myself, which means taking some time every day to move my body (sometimes just a good stretch, a backbend, and a walk) and sit quietly, and most of all, to devote some time to doing nothing.

In closing, I'd like to offer this poem I wrote that was first published in the *Chariton Review* in 2016.

> I GO TO A SHALA
> I go to a shala
> to stand on one leg,
> plant inside
> winter's darker heart.
> I go to a shala to be
> for the sun, rise and fall
> with the burble
> of being—floorboards creak,
> a radiator clanks,
> we gaze at the steadily falling
> snow. Balance, our desire—
> stalk to sunflower's eye—
> black light
> in summer's bay—
> How to divine
> this wobbling, what is
> before and beyond
> inherited traits—

I go to flow in unknown straits,
flip and twist
until we come ashore—
to raise our necks, listen
to what we need to say
then lie down and die for a while.

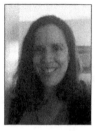

Kathleen Kraft is a writer, yoga teacher, and an editor at Yoga International. Her chapbook, *Fairview Road*, was published by Finishing Line Press, and her work has appeared in many journals, including *Five Points, Sugar House Review, Gargoyle*, and *The Satirist*.

# BLOODLESS WOUNDS

## *Elliot Kesse*

I often talk about my past life and my current life. Not in some existential or metaphysical sense. I'm an atheist. I don't have a need for any of that. But all in this lifetime, two years turned me into a different person. Almost everything has changed: my friends, my support network, what I'm willing to accept (or tolerate), how I behave—it's all completely different. While a lot of things played a part, without yoga this dramatic change wouldn't have been possible. It removed barriers that prevented me from receiving the benefits or fully feeling the effects of all the other pieces.

## I Never Just Fit

It's amazing how normal struggling can seem. When you've never known any different, you don't always know life can be different. Normal as stress and misery is just what you know.

I was always the weird one. I never quite fit in even in groups where I should. I was weird in my family. I wasn't quite like any of my friends. I just didn't seem to have a place in the world. I was the fat one, the awkward one, and then the chronically ill one. Whatever it was, there was always something other people had to tolerate in order to have me around. I never just fit.

"You're so weird. Why are you always reading? Go play with your cousins!"

It was so obvious to me that I kept who I really was a secret. I didn't mention hurtful things that would happen, even though I should've been screaming them. My constant fear of being abandoned, of being shunned, of being excluded, meant I knew I needed to keep secrets. I needed to play the part of who everyone thought I was and who they wanted me to be. There was no way I could show them who I really was. Because obviously no one would want to be around the real me.

## A New Life Seeps In

But I had no way to put this into words. No way to acknowledge this was my reality. I was essentially operating in survival mode. *Just do what you need to so everyone doesn't leave you.* When you're just trying to survive, when you're desperately clinging to a barely held together reality, you live in a world of stress and sadness. But I didn't know this. Or, rather, I couldn't know this. I couldn't have survived if I knew there was another reality possible. That became abundantly clear, whether I wanted it to or not, once I was exposed to bits and pieces of my new life. And once I was aware of it, I couldn't ignore it; no matter how hard I tried, physically, my own body wouldn't let me ignore it.

When I was a child, I had to be the good one, the responsible one. I had to get good grades and never get in trouble. I worked, was on academic team and in band. The chronic pain and illnesses started showing vague signs in my childhood. But I was told to behave and to stop looking for attention.

"No one wants to be around a whiner."

By the time I was an adult, I had learned that the only way I could be in relationships was if I didn't ask for too much, didn't take up too much space. I would only be kept around if I wasn't a burden on anyone else.

"You're always asking for help. You're selfish!"

The day I left my home, I hadn't planned on leaving. But I couldn't breathe. That's not a metaphor or exaggeration. The weight of my past life had become so much I physically could not will my body to bring air into my lungs any longer. My throat was closing shut. I had to get out of that house right away. And I did. I grabbed a few essentials— some clothes, my meds—and I left. The few times I returned to get an item I needed, absolute panic would set in. One of the last times I was there, I experienced so much panic being in that house again. I was racing around trying to get some of my things before a panic attack set in. It seemed so chaotic and loud even though I was alone and it was silent. When I made it back to my car after collecting a few things, my first thought was, "I made it. I made it out. And I never have to go back again." I just sat there, in my driver's seat, crying for I don't know how long.

## Invisible Trauma

We often think of trauma and abuse as major, catastrophic events that destroy a person in one fell swoop, leaving them lifeless, bruised, and bloodied on the ground. It's only trauma if it's visible. Trauma that bites at your ankles and leaves marks only within the body is invisible and, as such, doesn't exist. At best, we're discouraged from talking about it but more often than not, we're shamed for wanting it acknowledged, for wanting better, different. And because it often involves those closest to us, we have that extra weight of shame pushed on us to carry around because calling out the toxic behavior means violating this sacred expectation that family, whether genetic or through a marriage license, comes first no matter what.

"I'm only telling you this because I care about you."

"Family is all that matters. Your friends don't care about you like I do."

I also didn't know that people who loved you could also abuse you. I thought if someone loves you, you just had to accept everything they did. Because they love you and they're doing everything out of love, and you should just appreciate it and be happy with that.

But the first and longest relationship you have isn't with family or friends. It's with yourself. And your body is how you experience your life. It's how you experience the world. If you're not at home in your body, if you're not comfortable in your body, you can't trust anything. Every sensation is questioned, every sensation is a possible threat. You're never not on guard.

## We're Taught Not to Trust Ourselves

In general, American society actively encourages us to disconnect from our bodies, to not trust ourselves. This was true in the working-class culture I grew up in. Be strong, don't complain, work harder, defer to authority, and pull yourself up by your bootstraps. As my chronic illnesses progressed, the idea that my body wasn't to be trusted, that I didn't know what was going on with myself, was constantly reinforced by every medical professional I had the misfortune of interacting with. It was yet another layer telling me I was wrong, and I couldn't trust myself.

"Good news! Your results are within range. There's nothing wrong with you. You're probably just depressed."

So I found myself in relationships where my well-being wasn't a consideration, where, if I didn't sacrifice my own health to appear "normal" or how others thought I should be, I was shamed. It was very clear that most of my relationships could only exist if I kept large parts of myself hidden, if I didn't talk about myself too much. This inevitably led to relationships where I ceded control of myself and my life to others, and of course, the wrong people were more than willing to take control for me. I was willing to do anything to make others happy, but that's not how abusive relationships work. Nothing you do can ever be enough, nothing can ever be right. You'll always be wrong.

"You're not hungry. You don't need to eat that."

"You're not sick. You don't need a wheelchair."

I was a chronic and unquestioning people pleaser. People pleaser. That sounds like such a good thing. Like, who wouldn't want to please people? Why wouldn't you want to make people happy? But it sets you up for exhaustion and sadness, and primes you to become a victim, taken advantage of, intentionally or not, by others.

"It doesn't matter if you're uncomfortable. You're being selfish. They asked you to do it."

## Finding Myself in Yoga

The first time I did yoga was in college. I didn't really know much about it other than it was different than anything people I knew were doing and, probably because I always felt so different, I gravitated toward anything I perceived as different. Maybe I'd fit there. I don't remember much about that class other than it was in a school gym after classes. Over the next fifteen or so years I did yoga off and on. Every time, I fell in love with it and how it made me feel. I was mostly focused on the physical, thinking yoga would make my body smaller and more acceptable. But I always noticed how it changed the way I felt in my body. I couldn't put words to it, but I felt strength in my body that I couldn't find otherwise. Eventually, because it made me feel in a way I couldn't find the ability to feel with anything else, I started going more frequently. I eventually discovered meditation and pranayama. Between the depression, anxiety, and pain, things started to shift.

Without much intent or awareness in the beginning, the importance of a physical practice started to wane. I still did asana several times a week, but it wasn't my goal, it wasn't where I found my strength. I began instead to find strength in my breath.

I was hiding in the stillness, in the inhales and exhales, the pauses between the poses. For the first time in my life, I met myself. And, much to my surprise, I liked myself.

Strange things start to happen when you sit with yourself. I slowly began to realize how much knowledge I was holding within my body. I started to realize that, by simple virtue of being, I had value. I didn't need to prove myself, I didn't have to be useful, I didn't have to do anything in order to be worthy of love and respect and acceptance. I just had to be.

"You are worthy."

Yoga brought a new relationship with myself, but it also brought lots of other new relationships within a new community. Previously, I had always felt that I had to hide who I was in order to be tolerated by others. If those "undesirable" parts came out, others would be uncomfortable, and I'd be abandoned. The other's comfort always being more important than my well-being. If I wasn't useful, then I was a burden, and why would anyone want me around? I had never before been surrounded by people who made me feel accepted and welcome simply for being myself. I'd never felt like I could walk away from people who made me feel less than for any reason. I didn't know I could say it was unacceptable to be treated that way.

"I deserve to be loved as a whole person."

One of the biggest things that I discovered were boundaries. Despite my therapist mentioning them over and over, I never understood them. It's impossible to when you don't have any understanding of your innate value. When she would talk about boundaries, I thought they sounded horrible. I couldn't imagine anything worse than telling someone that I had an expectation or need and that it should be respected even if they didn't like it. That would hurt their feelings. I should just do whatever they wanted to make them happy, regardless of what it meant to my mental and physical health and safety. That was the only way to make sure they wouldn't abandon me, that I wouldn't be too much of a burden on them, that I wouldn't make them too uncomfortable. Over the years that I saw her, I'm fairly certain that I rolled my eyes every time my therapist mentioned boundaries. It wasn't until I stumbled on a little bit of self-worth in the stillness of yoga that I began to understand what boundaries were and why I needed them.

It's not unusual for someone to ask why when I tell them that meditation changed everything for me. I tell them it was because I'm the one who has to sit with me during meditation so no one else's opinion matters. Until they're the ones who have to sit within me for those ten minutes or an hour or whatever, until they have to swim through the voices in my head and feel the emotions in my body, until they're the ones who have to do that, their opinion doesn't matter. And because no one else can do that, no one else knows what's best for me.

"I'm the only one who can take care of myself."

Another thing yoga taught me was that none of us are perfect. My idea of abuse was that it was always done by someone who was bad or evil. Good people, nice people, caring people don't abuse. But that's simply not true. Otherwise good people abuse others all the time. Whether it's because it's "normal" behavior for them and they're repeating the only behavior they've seen, or whether it's because the coping skills they learned to survive when they needed them have become toxic and problematic now that they're out of that situation. Whatever the reason, the abusers in my life, and many others I've seen and heard about, aren't always evil. They aren't abusive all of the time.

## Owning My Shit

As my yoga practice developed, one thing that happened that no one seemed to be talking about was the revelation that I needed to work on myself the same way I expected others to work on themselves. If I expected others to "own their shit," I needed to "own my shit." I needed to recognize that my own behavior could be toxic to myself and others. And I needed to put the work in to acknowledge and address those behaviors.

Again, it was within the stillness of yoga that I realized this and was able to start working on myself. There is no end to this work. I will never be perfect. But I will show up and continue to "own my shit" every day. I won't allow the past to continue to have control over me by bringing the bad into the present. The past happened. I survived. I learned. I'm growing. Every. Day.

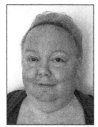

Elliot Kesse is a fat, white, atheist, agender spoonie who strives to create safe spaces for joyful movement and practical stillness for all humans. They founded change.yoga and are anti-diet and pro-self-empowerment. They live, practice, and teach with several chronic physical and mental illnesses including autoimmune and endocrine diseases, depression, anxiety, and suicidal thoughts. Visit them at www.change.yoga.

# YOGA JEANS

## *Celisa Flores*

I was four years old in 1985. The year before, my grandmother, my primary caregiver, had died suddenly. I, along with my siblings and cousins, had been raised by my maternal grandmother while our parents worked. My memories of my grandmother are limited, but my general sense from that time was of feeling safe, protected, carefree, and confident. After her rapid decline, my parents were tasked with finding care at least for me, the youngest of three, since I wasn't in school yet. My father mostly worked nights in an effort to balance the childcare duties. My mother—in grief, in law school, and employed—had night shift with us.

Being with my parents as full-time parents was an adjustment for everyone. They were burdened with work and school and responsibilities that my grandmother had not been, and this likely made parenting a sensitive child even more of a challenge. One example of this challenge came when I chose to be vegetarian at age four, which was difficult to accommodate when being shifted around to babysitters and school. Later in life, I learned that I had multiple undiagnosed severe food allergies and sensitivities, so many foods left me feeling unwell. Food allergies were hardly on anyone's radar or even acknowledged at that time, so the message I most consistently received was that I was being dramatic, that I was attention seeking, or that I was being manipulative. My four-year-old mind's interpretation of those messages was that I was wrong, that I couldn't trust my body's signals, and that I was an unreliable source for understanding my own experience.

A bar review course recommended my mother try yoga to manage stress, and not wanting to miss any recommendation that may help her pass the bar, she took me along. Yoga was offered at one location in my hometown: the retired teachers' association. The class was taught by an older gentleman who showed up most days in jeans, a T-shirt, and socks. Most people wore sweatpants and brought along a towel to delineate their space or just practiced on the musty carpet of the dimly lit church. Following asana practice, we practiced silent meditation, and I slipped into this easily—one of the few times I welcomed silence.

We attended this hatha based yoga practice several nights weekly for several months while my mother was studying for the bar, and I also practiced rolling around in postures at home. Yoga was fun and silly for me and a space where I felt some sense of mastery over my own body. And I liked spending time with the retired teachers who reminded me of my grandmother I had recently lost.

## Escape Routes

By age eleven, I had struggled for years with depression and intense anxiety, with feeling disconnected from my own body, and feeling like an imposter in a school for gifted children. I had lived in the shadow of my brother two years older than me, whom I always thought of as the smart and compliant one. With a sense that I couldn't fill those expectations, I chose the path of quiet rebellion and was drinking alcohol and smoking cigarettes at school in fifth grade. Socially, I was often inappropriate, abrasive, and lacked the skills to connect in any healthy way. I was friends with the outcasts, and we made sure to do everything we could to cause trouble without too much consequence.

Finding alcohol and marijuana in elementary school created distance between myself and my overwhelming feelings but also from my healthier coping strategies, like yoga. I continued my practice to a much lesser degree, and this was devastating for my connection with my body. I got to a place where my perceived faulty interpretations made me just wish my body would disappear, or at least submit to my will. In a time before the internet, I spent my time looking at medical dictionaries to learn about the different types of eating disorders. I remember reading that a possible side effect of bulimia is tooth decay, and that was the deciding factor for me; I "chose" anorexia.

After years of training as an eating disorder therapist, I now know that while I may have "chosen" to start with anorexia, there is very little willpower involved in sustaining an eating disorder. Brain scans of people with anorexia show variance in brain function and volume as well as production, availability, and use of neurochemicals, including oxytocin, often referred to as the love chemical.[38] My brain is different than that of someone who has never had anorexia. And although the research is often inconclusive about these differences as cause or consequence, it's hard to imagine that anyone could override our most human instinct to survive without some brain variance.

I got through most of high school active in my eating disorder and active in little else. In my eating disorder, I developed a strong aversion to any type of exercise. I continued to practice hatha yoga intermittently but never to the point that I would break a sweat. When I did occasionally find myself back in meditation practice, I would notice a nagging voice reminding me how much I was damaging my body.

So, at fifteen, I made the first of many efforts to approach sobriety and even eat one meal a day without seeking support, because that had felt like such a foreign concept for so much of my life. Though my distorted

38. Guido Frank, Jeremy R. Reynolds, Megan E. Shott, Leah Jappe, Tony T. Yang, Jason R. Tregellas, and Randall C. O'Reilly, "Anorexia Nervosa and Obesity Are Associated with Opposite Brain Reward Response," Neuropsychopharmacology 37, no. 9 (May 2012): 2031–46, https://doi.org/10.1038/npp.2012.51; Walter H. Kaye, Julie L. Fudge, and Martin Paulus, "New Insights into Symptoms and Neurocircuit Function of Anorexia Nervosa," *Nature Reviews Neuroscience* 10, no. 8 (August 2009): 573–584, https://www.nature.com/articles/nrn2682; Elizabeth A. Lawson, Laura M. Holsen, McKale Santin, Erinne Meenaghan, Kamryn T. Eddy, Anne E. Becker, David B. Herzog, Jill M. Goldstein, and Anne Klibanski, "Oxytocin Secretion Is Associated with Severity of Disordered Eating Psychopathology and Insular Cortex Hypoactivation in Anorexia Nervosa," *The Journal of Clinical Endocrinology & Metabolism* 97, no. 10 (October 2012): 1898-1908, https://doi.org/10.1210/jc.2012-1702.

thoughts remained, I thought I was in recovery from my eating disorder. I was not near weight restoration, nor had menstruation resumed, but in my teenage mind, I was fine, great even. Now, as a therapist who specializes in working with eating disorders, if I had met my younger self, I would have recommended hospitalization for her.

## Unexpected

Months into my early recovery efforts, I found out there was another reason for the lack of consistent menstruation: I was pregnant at sixteen. Prior to the confirmed pregnancy, I had been pretty certain that my fertility was too compromised to be a concern. When I went for my first obstetrics visit, my doctor told me he wouldn't see me again for three months because he didn't think I could sustain a pregnancy beyond the first trimester due to being so underweight.

I went home and sobbed, big, heaving sobs, feeling betrayed by my body. Then, in a moment of silent exhaustion, when coming back to my breath felt like all I had left, I considered that maybe I had been the one betraying my body. I had wanted for so long to be invisible, to make even my most basic needs invisible, that I lost track of what those needs even were.

I made the decision that I was going to do everything I could to sustain the pregnancy. I reminded myself that I could always go back to my eating disorder later. As unhealthy as it seems in retrospect, that was an important piece for me to be able to come back to when I was overwhelmed by my distorted thoughts. I knew that the longer I could challenge the behaviors, the better off I would be and the better the outcome of my pregnancy. Pregnancy was the first time in a very long time I had felt calm and comfortable in my own body, so I did my best to make the most of the time. While I sorted out my next step, I read everything I could on pregnancy, started eating dairy and poultry, and practiced from books I found on prenatal yoga. I cried every time I ate animal products through all of my pregnancy and nursing but persisted all the same.

Five days past my expected delivery date, in record-breaking heat, more than double the weight I had been right before pregnancy, I was told that my twenty-two inch, almost nine-pound baby was a boy.

## Keep Pushing

As a single parent, I stayed busy, taking my little one to college with me, to volunteer positions, and of course, to yoga classes. When he stayed with his grandparents, however, I did not know what to do with myself. I had spent so long in meditation working on acceptance and non-attachment, yet I found it such a challenge to be without my son. I was filled with so much fear and anxiety about being apart from him, and those feelings were only compounded by my own experiences of grief and loss and heartbreak and trauma. So nights he was away, I went back to my childhood coping skill: I drank. A lot.

During that time, I had found a studio that offered a heated vinyasa that ran anywhere from ninety minutes to two hours, depending on how the instructor felt. This studio was much different than the yoga experience of my childhood. Though it was a great studio, there was certainly no encouragement to check our egos at the door. I went no matter what and there was a sense that we should try to "push through." On good days, I felt so strong, grounded, and empowered there. On days I was sick or hungover, I felt I deserved to suffer, and I used asana practice to punish myself. I continued this cycle for years until finally, at twenty-seven, after a night of especially excessive drinking for Valentine's Day, I decided I was done drinking to escape my feelings.

I went to yoga, I went to therapy, I practiced breathwork and meditation daily. There were still days that were heartbreaking, soul crushing, and devastating. I took up sewing and baking and volunteered in my son's class. I worked full time as a therapist and enrolled in a weekend doctoral program that was five hours away. Instead of escaping with alcohol and my eating disorder, I was escaping with "busyness." Despite my training as a therapist, I felt so unprepared to deal with my feelings without trying to escape.

After careful consideration and deliberation for months, I decided to move to Orange County, where my doctoral program was based. This meant leaving the support system we had and building our new community. My old fears of being an imposter and of my son being away from me came back with a vengeance.

Daytime yoga classes in Newport Beach meant overhearing discussions of nannies, full price yoga clothes, and taking $4,000 teacher training for the sake of "being the best in class." I had been a single parent my entire adult life. I had only ever shopped at thrift stores and clearance racks for my clothes and had mostly taken three dollar yoga classes in gymnasiums or empty churches where we followed along with yoga cassette tapes in unison. The distance between my experience and the Newport dream made me homesick and long for the days of yoga teachers who showed up in jeans.

Between writing my dissertation on mindfulness training for students, I managed to continue yoga classes and stumbled into a Kundalini class that became my yoga crush. I felt I had finally experienced the yoking of mind-body. Though Kundalini involves breath and asana practice similar to my previous experiences with hatha and vinyasa yoga, there is a different sense of internal focus, with the goal of awakening internal energy. This practice helped me find a new yoga community, and a small hand-poked Om tattoo inside my arm reminded me to refocus when my attention wandered from my own practice. I finished school with certifications in Mindfulness-Based Stress Reduction and Yoga for Psychologists that I had managed to work in as components of my dissertation

Though we had planned to return to our hometown when I finished school, my son was already having an amazing high school experience that couldn't be replicated in our hometown. I had found work before even finishing school, working as a therapist in an eating disorder program, one area I had never even considered working in during my training. I loved the challenge of working with people recovering from eating disorders and addiction, and I was able to share my training in mindfulness and meditation.

## Ahimsa

Then, two days before my birthday, I won a partial scholarship for a yoga teacher training at YogaWorks. It had been a dream of mine for years to complete a teacher training, but it seemed so out of reach. YogaWorks is a national chain of yoga studios started in 1987, and the training was comprehensive, organized, and focused on the parts of yoga that were important to me. I had already trained as a birth doula and being able to add empowerment tools such as yoga for people in transition felt so in line with my purpose.

On the morning of our prenatal yoga training, I was involved in a major hit and run car accident. My car was totaled, and I had injuries that kept unfolding for months. I found myself so incredibly frustrated with my body, again. I had been using yoga asana to manage my stress and my insomnia, to fill my empty time, and as a source of community.

Though my practice waxed and waned, yoga had been the most consistent space I felt safe, and I was afraid to think how I might fill that gap if my practice changed. It wasn't until much, much later that I came to see this fear, as well as the fear of being away from my son and our community, as rooted in my efforts at attachment. My early loss left me in constant fear that anyone or anything I loved would be gone in an instant. The yogic concept of aparigraha is that of non-attachment, or non-grasping, not only to objects, but to ideas and relationships as well. This is a practice I still struggle with regularly and have come to remind myself that it is a practice.

After taking a short leave, I went back to take the required classes to complete teacher training. I decided to take a restorative class as my first class back with our prenatal trainer, whom I had missed a few weeks before. I explained that I would be modifying due to injuries from a recent accident. She paused to look me in the eyes and tell me that I should consider just lying on my mat, that it was ok to just nurture myself. I froze, eyes wide, breathless, as those words echoed in my head for what seemed like an eternity and reverberated in my soul like a Tibetan bowl. This was the permission I never realized I was waiting for and the first time since I was a child that I didn't feel like I should just "push through." This was the most important lesson in my teacher training.

Once I completed teacher training, I focused on creating accessible and trauma-sensitive yoga for people with eating disorders and those who were overcoming addiction in the program I was facilitating.

I offer postures modified for various body sizes, for those with no experience with yoga, and for those with medical recommendations to stay in seated or lying positions. I lead with props as primary and discuss the benefits of each posture. My own practice is very limited in asana practice; I move in ways that provide relief, and I always use props. My focus after multiple major car accidents has been on meditation and breathwork and learning and relearning the practices of ahimsa, or nonviolence, especially against myself, and aparigraha when facing losses, big and small.

I am fortunate enough to have worked for organizations that see the benefit of offering yoga practice as part of wellness and self-care. This has afforded me the opportunity to share my training in ways that are empowering and not cost prohibitive. I end every practice with the reminder that I am here only as a guide, that any moments of peace in the practice are always present and accessible at any time.

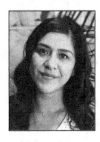

Celisa Flores began practicing yoga at age five, which served as a wellness tool throughout her life. Following her training as a therapist and, later, yoga and meditation teacher, these became empowerment skills she was able to share with clients, especially those struggling with eating disorders, addictions, and other mental health concerns.

Author photo by Alejandro Gomez.

# REBELLIOUS RESILIENCE

## Antesa Jensen

"You are disgusting."

It took twenty-four years for me to hear the thought loud enough to be broken by it. But once I heard it, I knew I had been an unconscious slave to it most of my life. The words in my head were spoken with a dysfunctional familiarity—as if this truth were an invisible limb I had been carrying around, whose main function was to observe my flaws and make sure I knew them anytime I got too confident.

## I Didn't Know My Body Belonged to Me

I was twelve the first time I was taken to get a colonic. I was told I had parasites and that my liver was overloaded and that I needed to cleanse my gut. The idea of having parasites inside of my body that I couldn't even see made my skin crawl. In that fear, knowing that I was dirty enough for dangerous bugs to live inside me, I definitely wanted to be clean.

I soon learned that it was about more than physical cleanliness, though, because when I outgrew spankings, I was sent to do enemas instead in a painful merging of metaphor and reality. If I had an attitude or didn't do my chores, I must be out of alignment. That meant there was rot in me and the irrigation of my bowels was meant to remove it. When I was particularly unruly, I was given a colonic.

I wasn't old enough to give my own consent: the colon therapist in the dingy basement wasn't deterred by that. He treated my preadolescent resignation and a signed document as permission, even though I was so clenched he needed extra lube to insert the tube in my anus.

## Take Your Power Back by Any Means Necessary

I remember being terrified that I might discover something gnarly about myself while lying there on the table with this older man's hands massaging my preteen belly. There's nothing quite as exposing as having your insides floating past you as they get examined by relative strangers.

This was not the first time I felt so betrayed—so violated at a cellular level—and it wasn't the last, but I remember deciding that evening that I would never share what was going on inside my body ever again. The risk was far too great.

But then something interesting happened. I immediately normalized the experience. I became addicted to herbal laxatives and enemas as a preventative measure against being taken to more colonics. I began to pride myself on what I knew about the gut, digestion, nutrition, and eventually epigenetics and the microbiome, emerging sciences at the time.

My compulsive and controlling behavior was never noticed because I was never skinny. My high intelligence and perceptivity, something I developed out of necessity during my childhood, and my overachieving perfectionist mentality were celebrated and rewarded by the people around me.

I was the one who had her shit together (literally and figuratively).

There's something instinctual that happens when, as young people, we feel our boundaries have been violated by those we trust. We choose (whether we're consciously aware of it or not) to repeat the violation willingly, sometimes repeatedly, to ourselves and with others, as a means to take our power back. An associative neural pathway gets created that says this abuse equals safety, and so we repeat it, over and over. Conversely, we begin to interpret safe things as dangerous and begin to reject the things we want most, convinced that having our needs truly met will result in harm. And this is how we attempt to convince ourselves of our own sovereignty.

## Learning to Trust Myself

I remember the first time one of my yoga teachers suggested we listen to our bodies in a vinyasa class. There were no mirrors in the room, and we were being invited to feel our own truth. I had started yoga haphazardly in my early twenties on the promise of a discount and a good workout, and it quickly became another thing I compulsively needed to perfect.

I was secretly willing her to come over and adjust my posture when she said it. Her validation that I was doing the posture correctly, as though there was only one expression of it that mattered, meant way more to me than listening to myself. Every external adjustment I received, and every confirmation I got that I was doing it right—"Beautiful Antesa, that's exactly it."—felt like a little win. I was feeding off of her recognition, because self-recognition was something I had in scarce supply.

I had a toxic relationship with precision. To me, precision was perfection. But over time, and in the absence of mirrors and in classes far too large for regular one to one adjustment, I had no choice but to eventually feel and listen to myself. I had to trust that I was doing it as right as I could.

And most importantly, I had to accept that this wasn't a performance, but rather, a practice. This was by far one of the most difficult elements of yoga for me.

I began to develop an appreciation for the wisdom of my body after the time I stretched backward into camel pose and immediately broke down into tears for no apparent reason. My teacher said to me, "Sometimes, the body just needs to cry." I never cried, but apparently sometimes my body just needed to. Like in all the heart-opening postures.

This was my first encounter with permission and self-trust.

And I had a long way to go.

## [Your] Truth Will Set You Free

It may come as no surprise that given my upbringing, and the sophisticated ways in which I adapted to my trauma, I had conflated my truth with facts and opinions. Any opportunity I had to gain mastery was taken on like the disciplined and lifelong student I was, but with an aim at getting it right. Along the way, I was also collecting opinions about things I believed to be wrong.

Because when I was right, I felt powerful. When I was wrong, I felt vulnerable. And being vulnerable was life-threatening.

The thing about truth is that it exists outside of right and wrong. It just is. It's an all-encompassing revealing of the present moment. Nothing more, nothing less. It is inherently value neutral.

In order to access that truth, I had to be present, which means I needed to let go of my past and stop worrying about the future long enough to do that in body, mind, and spirit.

This was not an easy task for me because I was so attached to being right.

And so I just decided that there were right ways to feel and wrong ways to feel and I only allowed myself to feel the right things.

Although my mindset embraced failure, failure was only acceptable so long as I was a safe distance ahead of the pack or otherwise very well hidden where no one could see me stumble.

Eventually, I reached a point where maintaining this lifestyle was no longer possible. The anxiety of always needing to be ten steps ahead and right all the time was destroying my sleep, my health, and my relationships. I was starting to crumble.

It was at this point that I made two important choices that forever changed my life: I began meditating, and I hired a life coach who had a knack for mothering and building nurturing relationships that was so profound it almost repulsed me. That repulse was my cue that she had something I probably had no idea I needed.

The purpose of the meditation practice was simply to feel. The focus was on noticing physical sensations as they arose, and the practice was for fifteen minutes a day. It seemed like no big deal, but of course during my first attempt I cried.

It seemed I had a pretty hefty backlog of tears stored in my body, but at that point I understood—thanks to the grace of my yoga teachers—that sometimes the body needs to cry. And so I let myself unravel, slowly at first, and then all at once.

## You Don't Need a Reason to Feel Your Feelings

I felt ashamed, embarrassed, and confused. Where were these tears even coming from? Why were they happening? I was desperate to find a reason but continued to come up empty.

My coach taught me an important lesson during this period that has become the cornerstone of the work I now do with my own clients: we don't need to have a reason to feel our feelings, and our feelings are real and very much a part of our truth.

It hadn't occurred to me up until this point that my power didn't come from being right; my power came from being honest.

About how I feel.

About how I have been impacted.

About what I desire in my life.

Where rightness was once my performance, radical honesty quickly became my practice.

Developing the capacity to feel and subsequently identify and share our feelings, needs, and desires—both physical and emotional—and to express them truthfully, is the foundation of yoga.

In the *Yoga Sutras of Patanjali*, Sutra 36 says "To one established in truthfulness, actions and their results become subservient."[39]

What this is suggesting is that when we live a life grounded in truth-telling, we are aligning ourselves in the present moment, and all things that once required effort become easy.

I call this emotional biohacking.

39. Sri Swami Satchidananda, trans., *The Yoga Sutras of Patanjali*. *13th ed. (Yogaville, VA: Integral Yoga Publications, 2008), 131.*

# Holding Space

Learning to feel my feelings was the first of many steps toward healing my relationship with myself, and eventually, my relationships with others, even those who had hurt me. This is a reality I never even thought would be possible. And I never would've been able to successfully do that if I hadn't had many teachers and mentors hold space for that to happen for me.

Holding space means listening without a need to respond, validate, relate to, analyze, or otherwise process what was shared. It's listening without judgment, agenda, or predetermined destination.

This sort of listening requires a high level of both empathy, awareness, and experiential training. To hold space in this way is a deeply vulnerable act. And it's a skill set that is both desperately needed and sorely missing in most environments, especially our most intimate relationships.

We are so trained to create connection by processing our feelings with one another, but what we don't tend to realize is that processing with friends or family can easily prevent us from the deeper healing we most need, because most friends (and our families, peers, and even our significant others) don't have the training to execute this effectively.

In most cases, healing, transmutation, and alchemy (converting wounds into blessings, for example) are expansive in nature, and in order to expand, we need space.

What took me years to understand was that those who caused me harm couldn't offer that kind of emotional support to me because they never got that training. They lacked the capacity to do that for me when I needed it most because they couldn't even do it for themselves. How could I fault them for something they never had the resources to know they needed? Understanding this reality provided me with a lot of relief.

Healing, however, does not just come from understanding. It comes from feeling those forgotten emotions we left at "the scene of the crime" all the way through until you get to compassion and ultimately forgiveness. Understanding the perspective of those who hurt me is not what healed me of my pain. It was in diving deep into feelings I once instinctively had shut down, increasing my capacity to feel those feelings, and then recognizing all of the times I also did not hold space—for myself and for others—when it mattered most because I also lacked that capacity. And then forgiving myself for that and actively learning another way of being that was more kind.

One of the most beautiful ways this has actualized in my life is that I now get to show other people how to hold space by listening to them as they move all the way through this process. And it has helped me manifest the profound and connected relationships that I'd spent years longing for. Yes, I also learned boundaries that have proven priceless in my growth, but my ability to listen is what has nurtured our collective growth.

One of my favorite ways to hold space for others when they have so bravely shared their truth with me is to say, "Thank you for sharing that with me."

Because in reality, anytime anyone shares a truth, what they're really doing is offering a gift.

## Rebellious Alchemy

A key element I attribute to much of my success, and ultimately healing, is my defiant streak. The unembodied, yet resilient, little girl who chose self-preservation and who once felt at odds with her family wasn't all wrong. In healing and embodying the part of me that made those choices because I believed I was disgusting, I got to make ample use of the parts that have made me so successful now, in my personal life and relationships, as well as in my business. Because the current model for most is to avoid, deny, and numb out our problems, my defiance helped me take those necessary first steps toward another—healthier—way of being.

The subconscious mind is insidious, which means that there will always be, no matter how far along on the path we are, compelling reasons to not dig deeper into our own psyches. We create sophisticated forms of resistance in order to stay safe automatically and can easily find ourselves out of alignment, especially during the earlier stages of a path of inner inquiry when we still don't have enough discernment to trust ourselves. It's an act of rebellious alchemy to transmute our wounds into the innate gifts that have been waiting for us all along.

It's rebellious because we live in a world where the mass majority are still running away. To lean in when things get tough requires grit, commitment, devotion, and faith that something better that we can't yet see MUST exist on the other side of suffering even though the pull is to stay comfortable and ignorant. It's alchemy because energy cannot actually leave our bodies—we can't expel our pain or put it on someone else; it can only change form. We must be willing to consider that what is causing us the most pain has the potential to bring us the most joy in order for this process to take place.

It's my personal experience that success in life, as well as in business, stems from believing in our own product—ourselves—unequivocally. In order to believe in ourselves, we must trust ourselves. In order to trust ourselves, we must learn to listen to ourselves.

I work with powerhouse trailblazers with an entrepreneurial spirit who—like me—have struggled to trust themselves fully, feel comfortable embracing their emotional experience, and thoroughly heal past trauma so that they can finally bring their voices into the world and live as the fullest expression of themselves. I work with them in creating their own path of rebellious alchemy so that they can claim their birthright of offering their innate gifts to the world.

Because in order to make an impact, we must first recognize that we are impacted.

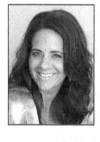

Antesa Jensen is an emotional intelligence expert specialized in evoking and conjuring the genius in others, and then resourcing them with the necessary tools to perpetually actualize their innate human potential. She works with individuals and businesses in cultivating these skills through keynote speeches, bespoke transformational experiences, and one to one coaching. Learn more at antesajensen.com.

Author photo by Wendy Yalom Photography.

# THE ALCHEMY OF TRAUMA

## *Sanaz Yaghmai*

It was July of 2012, my thirtieth birthday and two days before my wedding day. Friends and loved ones were gathered around the dining room table as I blew out the candles. My birthday wish? Complete my dissertation that year and live a lifetime of marital bliss with at least two children.

If only life were that simple. Over the course of the next few years I was faced with challenging yet divine experiences that directed me to delve inward and practice the art of surrender. I learned that socially constructed expectations set us up for disappointment. There is no linear path to life, for it carries natural ebbs and flows, like that of ocean waves; without them we become stagnant. Yoga eventually became a source which allowed me to flow through the tides without feeling like I'm drowning.

As I was going to sleep the night before my wedding, I felt a heavy, dark, and suffocating sensation weighing on my chest. My intuition was telling me to pull the brakes. During the six months of wedding planning I received subtle messages from my intuition trying to redirect me, but I ignored her, as I was too focused on my end goal: married by thirty, two children by thirty-four, run a thriving psychology practice, live happily ever after.

As an Iranian American female immigrant from a middle-class family, I felt this was the most revered path to success. My perception of success and happiness was shaped by sociocultural conditioning that seeped deep into my identity and had become *my* dreams. Approval from others laid the foundation for "success," and fitting into neatly labeled boxes was the goal.

Three months after a beautiful wedding we started discussing divorce. Being a therapist, I paid close attention to my emotional state and noticed feelings of fear, guilt, shame, and inadequacy running through every fiber of my being. I was slipping into a depression and needed a safe space to share my fears as I navigated this potential divorce. I began seeing a therapist in November of 2012.

A year later the marriage was over. Divorced at thirty-one with a dissertation still looming over my head. My world was turned upside down, and I had no blueprint on how an Iranian woman in her early thirties navigates life after divorce. Although I come from a divorced family, my mother committed to twenty-one years of marriage before she decided to leave. My parents worked on sustaining their "happily-ever-after," enduring interpersonal hardships. But at what cost? With such an abrupt divorce, my path fed into the narrative that I was "less than," not "good enough," a "failure," and a "quitter." These words dominated my inner dialogue. Fortunately, I had overwhelming support from family and friends, I was told I was brave, that I was strong. Nonetheless, it didn't loosen the grip of shame.

## Critical and Compassionate Self-Inquiry

I often told my clients that coming to therapy is a courageous act of strength and self-love, but I had no idea how much courage it actually took until I was in the client's seat. Tears flowed as I opened the gates to a sea of repressed thoughts. So focused on external validation, I had lost touch with my core. Does a divorced woman in her midthirties with no children represent inadequacy? Does her worth diminish? I am worthy, as I am, without being a wife and mother, right?

Together with my therapist, I began to critically assess the shaping of my identity, peeling away the layers of sociocultural conditioning while reconnecting with my core self. In hindsight, my journey into yoga began in therapy through the practice of *svadhyaya* (self-study) and *ahimsa* (non-harming). Mindfully and compassionately, we worked at unraveling externally sourced beliefs from my own. I cried in that room every week for almost a year. It was overwhelming and frightening to question my core with no idea where I was headed and confused over my values. Painful and scary as it was, I began to reclaim power over my thoughts and started rewriting my narrative.

My experience of crying was different in therapy; the tears resided deeper within. I could hear and feel the thumping of my racing heart, I sweat profusely, and my entire body trembled, sometimes for the full hour. The words I uttered had an immediate impact on my physiology. I left each session feeling physically and emotionally exhausted with a lingering headache. I often needed to sleep afterwards. Although my mind was being tended to in therapy, slowly liberating me from the constraints of expectations and binary thinking, it was creating physiological responses that needed attention.

One morning I awoke with an odd, powerful intuitive message to get my thyroid tested despite never having thyroid issues. Sure enough, tests revealed I had developed an autoimmune disease of the thyroid known as Hashimoto's. A condition common in women, and often triggered by stress, it carries a host of symptoms including depression, anxiety, fatigue, brain fog, joint pain, forgetfulness, and dry skin, to name a few. This diagnosis was pivotal; it was evidence of the intricate powers of the mind-body interplay. I decided that it was time to tend to my needs on a more holistic level. Upon researching both the benefits and different branches of yoga, I felt a pull toward Kundalini yoga. I had never practiced any form of physical yoga and was intrigued by its blend of *mantra* (chanting), *dhyana* (meditation) and *pranayama* (breathwork) into the physical practice of postures and movement, the *asana*.

# Kundalini Yoga

Therapy had me in my head and yoga brought me into my body. Slowly but surely, I led myself into my self, flowing through the process of *self-unfoldment*.

My first experience of the physical practice of yoga was the start of my spiritual journey. I experienced an awakening of my entire being: the spaces between my mind, body, and spirit entered my consciousness. Kundalini yoga enabled me to viscerally access my inner strength by attuning to my soul. I began to learn a new language, that of the body, communicating with her through pranayama, meditation, asana, and mantra. Through controlling my breath, mind, physical body, and voice, I was controlling the flow of *prana* (energy/life force). Accessing and igniting these tools allowed for moments of bliss, grief, anger, and everything in between.

During my first class I was uncontrollably crying on my mat, a cathartic release of intense anger and guilt from holding on to self-hatred. As I moved from fast-paced movements to complete stillness I felt the discomfort dissipate. My controlled breathwork regulated my senses. Through the chants I felt emotions arise that I didn't know existed; my voice would tremble. None of the feelings lingered, and by the end of class I was left with an overwhelming feeling of strength. I learned that I must move away from labeling feelings as "good" or "bad"; they simply *are*. Feelings carry wisdom, as they are conduits transmitting messages from the subconscious to the conscious. Once I came to this realization there was an energetic shift; I began to honor all feelings, particularly those that had been silenced and mislabeled. I began to notice their transient nature as their grip loosened within my body.

For two years I committed to weekly therapy and a consistent Kundalini practice. I was feeling well-resourced with innate and divine support. The clouds of depression and inadequacy were lifting. With a newfound resilience, I felt motivated to push forward in my career, which had been stagnant since the divorce. First, I completed my dissertation and graduated, and within a year I had accepted a clinical psychologist position at a male maximum-security prison in Northern California.

## Trauma Behind Prison Walls

Working with trauma survivors and marginalized communities was my passion. I felt particularly drawn toward the inmate population because of their deep enmeshment in a life of trauma. Not only physical, emotional, and intergenerational traumas, but those which reside in a life of poverty, discrimination, and systemic oppression from the prison industrial complex, all of which perpetuate vicious cycles of trauma.

Upon entering the prison walls on my first day, I noticed a heightened awareness of my physical body: its proximity to exit doors, the amount of space I take up, and a particular awareness of my femininity being surrounded by a hypermasculine energy. Each morning, I sought the tools of yoga (meditation and chanting) to maintain a sense of safety and strength. The practice helped create a barrier between myself and my surroundings, reminding me that I am capable, I can take up space, and I am worthy of being heard. It kept me committed to aligning my values with my purpose.

After a few sessions with my clients, I noticed a common theme: dysregulated breathing and either hyper- or hypoarousal. I decided to explore breathwork and mindfulness tools with those who seemed receptive to learn. Within six months, I had piqued the interest of enough clients to put in a request to start a yoga and meditation group. My plan was to co-facilitate with a yoga teacher, and I would teach meditation and mindfulness tools. The request was approved, and a dream was about to come true.

One day amidst the planning, an inmate approached me on the yard and asked some odd, detailed questions about my life. Although that was not uncommon, this felt different; he was too fixated on me, and I expressed this concern to my colleagues. Knowing that he was serving a life sentence for murdering his parents and girlfriend amplified my intuition, giving rise to an eerie sensation, to say the least. A few days later, as I was driving to work, I thought, "He's going to attack me today." I quickly shut that thought down and told myself not to be "so dramatic." I often told myself I was "too much," "too emotional," "too dramatic" when I thought or said things that seemed a little extreme. Shutting myself down had become a habit. I arrived at work and began walking along my usual path, through the prison yard, to get to my office.

The inmate ran up to me from behind. Seconds before he reached me, I turned around, at which point he started punching me in my face and head with both fists. I crouched to the ground and protected my face with my hands as he continued punching my head until the officers arrived. I was taken to the ER and treated for stitches to my eyebrow. I was left with a black eye and some cuts and bruises.

That was my last day at the prison. For months I experienced heightened paranoia, a fear of men, and a mistrust of authority. I didn't draw my curtains open for months because I thought "they" had men on the outside watching me. My fear and anger were directed more toward the system than the assailant. Why didn't I take my eerie feeling more seriously? Was it my fault? Was the assault planned? My gut was telling me that this was a retaliation for speaking up against and reporting suspicions of systemic injustices. A story for another time and a question for which I will likely never have an answer.

Despite my heart wanting to go back and start my yoga group, my body would not let me. Prison staff are exposed to shock trauma every day; during my eight months behind those walls, I experienced regular verbal abuse, sexual harassment, and witnessed extreme violence with a deadly weapon. There is also the burden of compassion fatigue and secondary trauma from witnessing the suffering; my morals and conscience were constantly being challenged. It was emotionally and spiritually draining.

Returning to the therapy room, I tried to process my symptoms, but the weight of my trauma lay heavy on my heart. Reliving old stories of being a quitter and "not enough," I had a desire to go back and disprove that narrative. I also knew better. My body knew this time, I needed yoga: to meditate, flow, and feel through the discomfort of my truths, to rebuild trust with my intuition.

# Trauma in the Body

I immersed into the research on healing trauma outside of the therapy room. Leading experts have highlighted the pathway in which traumatic memories become stored in the body. I learned that these memories are encoded through a different pathway than nontraumatic memories. A nontraumatic memory is stored in specific parts of the brain and recalled through a particular neural pathway, which registers it as an experience of the past. On the other hand, traumatic memory recall pathways don't process the same way. They bypass our "logical" and "reasoning" brain, thereby confusing the past with the present. In addition, they leave a *somatic imprint* where they are stored at the sensory level in our body's nervous system. We "remember" through visceral sensations, and our body either relives the memory through a sensory pathway or detaches entirely from the mind (dissociation).

When we aren't attuned to the mind-body interplay, we are more likely to feel a disconnect between the two. We may feel powerless or develop a fear of uncertainty around how our body will react, so we begin to avoid certain places, people, relationships, and situations. The responses are endless and unique to the survivor.

Traditionally, the Western approach to trauma places greater emphasis on the mind, overlooking lived experiences of the physical body. We now know that the body holds on to emotions that the mind cannot process; therefore, body-based practices that incorporate various forms of movement, ritual, creativity (self-expression through arts and music), and connection through community, offer a holistic approach that allows for a release of untapped, stagnant energies. The research and science were fascinating, and they gave me the motivation to immerse into yoga trainings and learn about its history, philosophy, and teachings.

The old me would have never thought of being a yoga teacher. Cultural messaging had informed me that an Iranian woman who has excelled in her education has no reason to teach yoga. This deeply rooted bias crept into my consciousness, and I felt terribly ashamed. Therein lies the practice of yoga: a disruptor, shift maker, and constant mirror. Yoga doesn't free you from suffering—it awakens you to it. Yoga makes room for pause and reflection, allowing the unconscious to become conscious and presenting a choice: either hold on to biases or lean into ugly truths and make room for growth. I chose to lean into my biases, examine their roots, and work to grow through them.

## Reintroducing My Self to the World

I completed a trauma-informed yoga (TIY) training followed by a 200-hour hatha yoga teacher training. By the end, I regained access to the empowering tools that Kundalini yoga awakened me to. With an emphasis on social justice, the trainings also revealed a harsh reality: my privilege had blinded me from the fact that recovery and healing require great social and financial privilege. With the social privilege of stable and supportive family and friends, as well as job security that afforded me the time *and* finances to focus on self-care, I had an abundance of "recovery privilege." To top it off, shortly after my teacher training, I received the news that I would begin to receive disability retirement as a result of the prison assault.

Upon receiving this news my *dharma* (purpose) was revealed. Moving forward, I would leverage my privilege in a way that creates room for others to have opportunity. I want to be of service while addressing health inequities in marginalized communities and normalize conversations around mental wellness and trauma. What is the purpose of awakening to our innate strengths in a life of solitude? For it is in community that we heal. This is yoga.

In 2019, I spent almost six months in Greece at a refugee camp with a predominantly Afghan community. During that time, I established a partnership with an NGO on the ground holding spaces centered around TIY for displaced women. I co-facilitated a TIY leadership training for women and led TI care trainings for humanitarian aid workers, examining the mind-body interplay while understanding secondary trauma and best practices for community care. The teachings of yoga led me down this path, inspiring me to take what I learned and make it accessible in oppressed communities in crisis.

Finally, to take this story full circle, I am nearing forty with no partner and no children, and yet I feel more whole than ever before—to me, this is success.

Yoga distances us from the constraints of social constructs and reconnects us to the ancestral knowledge of the body that is inaccessible by the mind. Our body and spirit deserve as much respect as our mind, and I've come to learn that psychology and yoga need one another when navigating challenging emotional states. Yoga has found a home in my body, when feelings of inadequacy, fear, or anxiety show up (as they often do) I trust that my higher Self will kindly listen and encourage me to flow through rather than hide. The more I commit to harnessing her voice on the mat, the quicker she shows up in moments of crisis off the mat. She reminds me that I am capable, I am courageous, and I am worthy.

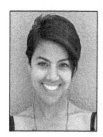

Sanaz Yaghmai, Psy.D is a Trauma-Informed Coach, yoga teacher, and doula. Formerly a psychologist, she has worked as a therapist in various communities over the last decade. Today, she is the founder of The Alchemy of Trauma, offering trauma-informed coaching and consulting services centered around post-traumatic growth, secondary trauma, and community building. In 2019, Sanaz implemented a trauma-informed yoga healing circle for displaced Afghan women and has continued supporting the community through online mentoring. She is also a board member of Refugym, a community-led NGO offering sports and wellness activities in refugee camps. Although she is "based" globally, Sanaz considers Los Angeles her home.

Author photo by Sarit Z Rogers.

# PART FIVE: REFLECTION QUESTIONS

- If I practice trusting myself …?
- What does it mean to belong?
- How does the practice of yoga remind me I have a place here and I belong?
- What does coming home to myself mean to me?

—Michelle C. Johnson

# CONCLUSION

So what's next?

We hope that the stories these contributors shared have inspired you to think critically and compassionately about the intersection of yoga, trauma, addiction, grief, loss, and resilience—to recognize that there is no one-size-fits-all approach to trauma, and that practices we may find useful ourselves might not be so useful for others (and vice versa).

We also hope these essays encourage you to seek out, build, and sustain strong, supportive communities that bolster the voices of people who have been marginalized: communities that listen to survivors, that recognize the complexity of everyone's experience, and that support post-traumatic growth, so that all of us may be encouraged to thrive and to celebrate that thriving.

Let's continue to listen. Let's continue to uplift one another. Let's keep the momentum going.

How we move forward and turn these conversations into action is up to us, and it can make a world of difference. Because in the end, each time a person heals and thrives, all of us heal and thrive.

# ACKNOWLEDGMENTS

Curating a collection like this takes time, patience, and a whole lotta love ... and we hope you feel that with every word you read.

We'd like to extend our sincere thanks and appreciation to all of the wise, brave, and beautiful voices in this book. Each contributor has generously offered their experience and insight to serve the collective healing process. We're grateful for the opportunity to have been invited intimately into their lives, work with them on the telling of their powerful stories, and share those stories with all of you.

Thanks to Angela Wix and Llewellyn for continuing to offer all of us as editors and writers the platform to publish this work over the last three volumes. *Embodied Resilience* has the opportunity to proudly stand on the shoulders of *Yoga and Body Image* as well as *Yoga Rising* due to the unwavering commitment from all of you at HQ.

We want to express our gratitude and love to our family and friends as well as the community partners, readers, and followers of our work over the years. Thank you for your love, support, and fierce commitment to us all.

# STAY IN TOUCH

We invite and encourage you to peruse the bios and websites of all of our contributors as a way to learn more about them and their work, as well as stay in touch. There are loads of amazing resources to glean from taking the time to access more information in this way.

Stay in touch with the Yoga and Body Image Coalition and access the free downloadable discussion guides associated with the previous anthologies by searching the links below.

Yoga and Body Image Coalition: http://ybicoalition.com
Facebook: https://www.facebook.com/ybicoalition
Instagram: http://www.instagram.com/ybicoalition
*Yoga and Body Image*: http://yogaandbodyimage.org
*Yoga Rising*: http://www.yogarisingbook.com/